来华留学生
中原中医药文化体验双语教程

朱剑飞 主编

山东科学技术出版社
·济南·

图书在版编目（CIP）数据

来华留学生中原中医药文化体验双语教程 / 朱剑飞主编 . -- 济南：山东科学技术出版社，2023.12
ISBN 978-7-5723-1560-2

Ⅰ.①来…　Ⅱ.①朱…　Ⅲ.①中国医药学—文化—汉、英　Ⅳ.R2-05

中国国家版本馆 CIP 数据核字 (2023) 第 015906 号

来华留学生中原中医药文化体验双语教程
LAIHUA LIU XUESHENG ZHONGYUAN ZHONGYIYAO
WENHUA TIYAN SHUANGYU JIAOCHENG

责任编辑：孙雅臻
装帧设计：侯　宇

主管单位：山东出版传媒股份有限公司
出 版 者：山东科学技术出版社
　　　　　地址：济南市市中区舜耕路 517 号
　　　　　邮编：250003　电话：（0531）82098088
　　　　　网址：www.lkj.com.cn
　　　　　电子邮件：sdkj@sdcbcm.com
发 行 者：山东科学技术出版社
　　　　　地址：济南市市中区舜耕路 517 号
　　　　　邮编：250003　电话：（0531）82098067
印 刷 者：山东蓝海印刷科技有限公司
　　　　　地址：山东省济南市高新区春田路南首 1 号
　　　　　　　　高新技术产业园 1 号厂房
　　　　　邮编：250101　电话：（0531）66725220

规格：16 开（170 mm×240 mm）
印张：13.5　字数：200 千　印数：1~2000
版次：2023 年 12 月第 1 版　印次：2023 年 12 月第 1 次印刷
定价：81.00 元

编委会

Editorial Board

序

　　中医药是中国的，又是世界的。中医药是中国的原创医学，又传播到 196 个国家和地区，为世界人类的健康做出了突出贡献。目前，中医药发展被提升为国家发展战略，进入了全方位、高质量发展的有利格局。中医药国际化迎来了历史上前所未有的战略机遇，在医疗服务、科研创新和文化传播等方面正加速协同推进，更大范围、更高水平、更深层次地走向世界。中医药国际化对于推动中西文化交流与对话，促进不同文明互学互鉴，增强民族文化自信心，增强中国软实力，提高中国话语权，为人类健康贡献中国智慧与中国方案，具有重要意义。

　　河南是中医药大省，是中华民族传统文化的发祥地，也是中医药学的重要发祥地。中医学的经典著作《黄帝内经》《伤寒杂病论》《神农本草经》主要在中原地区完成，中医药文化起源于中原，中医药大师荟萃于中原，中医药文化发达于中原，中医药巨著诞生于中原。河南作为中医药文化大省，理应在促进中医药国际传播和文化认同中起到示范和引领作用，以促进河南中医药文化传播，为健康中国贡献河南智慧和河南方案。

　　河南中医药大学是中国政府奖学金生培养高校，60 余年来，先后为50 余个国家培养留学生 3000 余名，在河南中医药对外开放中发挥着重要的示范和引领作用。近年来，学校在"国际知名，国内一流"办学实践中，来华留学生教育进入快速发展阶段，为学校"双一流"学科建设提供了有力的支撑。中医药高等教育是我国高等教育的重要组成部分，中医药

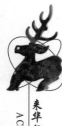

来华留学教育事业又是我国中医药高等教育的重要组成部分，发展中医药来华留学生教育事业依然是学校内涵建设的重要内容。

中原、中医、仲景是河南中医药文化的三大文化特色，做好中原、中医、仲景文化特色的挖掘、教学和国际传播，对于推动学校内涵建设、促进中医药开放发展意义重大。《来华留学生中原中医药文化体验双语教程》的编写在来华留学生教育方面做出了有益的探索，故欣然为序。

许二平

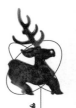

Foreword

Traditional Chinese medicine belongs to China and the world. Traditional Chinese medicine, an original form of medicine in China, has spread to 196 countries and regions and made outstanding contributions to the well-being of all people. At present, the development of traditional Chinese medicine has been promoted as a national development strategy and entered a favorable pattern of all-round and high-quality development. The internationalization of traditional Chinese medicine has ushered in unprecedented strategic opportunities in history. It is accelerating coordinated progress in medical services, scientific research innovation and cultural communication, and reaching out to the world on a larger scale and at a higher level. The internationalization of traditional Chinese medicine is of great significance to pushing cultural exchanges and dialogue between China and the west, promoting mutual learning and appreciation between different civilizations, strengthening national cultural confidence, enhancing China's soft power and discourse power, and contributing Chinese wisdom and scheme to human health.

Henan Province is a major province of traditional Chinese medicine, which is the birthplace of traditional Chinese culture, and also an important birthplace of traditional Chinese medicine. The classic works of traditional Chinese medicine such as *Huangdi Neijing* (*Yellow Emperor's Canon of Medicine*),

Shanghan Zabing Lun (*Treatise on Typhoid and Miscellanious Diseases*), and *Shennong Bencao Jing* (*Sheng Nong's Herbal Classic*) were mainly written in the Central Plains. The culture of traditional Chinese medicine originated in the Central Plains, where traditional Chinese medicine masters gathered and the culture of traditional Chinese medicine flourished. Furthermore, the great works of traditional Chinese medicine were born in the Central Plains. As a major province with traditional Chinese medicine culture, Henan Province should play a leading role in promoting the international dissemination and cultural identity of traditional Chinese medicine, so as to facilitate the spread of traditional Chinese medicine culture of Henan Province, and contribute wisdom and scheme with unique Henan characteristics to Healthy China Initiative.

Henan University of Chinese Medicine is a university with Chinese government scholarship for training overseas students. Over the past 60 years, Henan University of Chinese Medicine has cultivated more than 3,000 overseas students from more than 50 countries, playing an important demonstration and leading role in the opening up of Chinese medicine in Henan Province. In recent years, in the educational practice of being "internationally renowned and domestically first-class", the education of overseas students has entered a stage of rapid development, which provides strong support for the construction of "double world-class project" disciplines in the university. The higher education of traditional Chinese medicine is an important part of China's higher education, and the education of overseas students of traditional Chinese medicine in China is also an important part of China's higher education of traditional Chinese medicine. Thus, to develop the education of overseas students of traditional Chinese medicine in China is still an important part of the university's connotation construction.

Central Plains, traditional Chinese medicine and Zhongjing are the three cultural characteristics of traditional Chinese medicine culture of Henan Province. The excavation, teaching and international communication of the cultural characteristics of Central Plains, traditional Chinese medicine and Zhongjing is of great significance to the connotation construction of the university and the opening and development of traditional Chinese medicine. The compilation of *A Chinese-English Course on Traditional Chinese Medicine for Foreign Students in China* has made a beneficial exploration in the education of overseas students, so I'm glad to write the preface.

Xu Erping

前　言

　　语言教学和文化教学密不可分，语言是文化的载体。来华留学生到中国学习，除了需要掌握汉语的听说读写等基本技能外，还要了解具有中国特色的传统文化知识。只有以丰富的文化基础知识带动语言的学习，才能更好地完成学习任务。同时，文化体验通过提供真实文化环境引导学生亲身体验，能有效促进文化认同，提高文化教学效果。引导来华留学生深入学习中国、中原以及中医药文化，是中医药专业来华留学生培养的重要内容。因此，编写有利于"教"与"学"的中医药文化课体验教材势在必行。

　　目前，来华留学生文化教学存在教学内容趋同、教学模式单一、体验基地缺乏、教学主题缺乏特色等问题，严重制约了来华留学生对中国文化和中医药文化的认知和认同。为了解决以上问题，本书在编写过程中，围绕中医药文化，立足中原文化特色优势，着重突出了四大特色：双语特色、中医特色、中原特色、仲景特色。在突出特色的基础上，既强调中医技术的传播，又强调中医理论和文化的传播，更强调中原文化特色，为打造通俗易懂、图文并茂、中英对照、易于传播的中医药文化系列教材打下了坚实的基础。

　　本书共分为三章，按照中原、中医药、仲景文化模块编写，设计教学课时36学时，教师可以结合实际教学情况进行适当调整。同时，在每一个章节的教学内容后面都布置了实践活动和课后作业，建议教师可以根据地域文化特色，适当增加体验教学课时，加大文化实践活动教学比重，

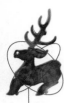

考虑理论教学和实践教学关系，重视文化教学师生双向交流，提高文化教学的针对性和趣味性。

　　本书的编者都是多年从事来华留学生汉语教学、文化教学、中医药专业教学的一线教师，教学经验丰富。尽管如此，由于来华留学生体验教学仍然处于探索阶段，教学大纲和教学内容校级差异显著，编者水平有限，本书肯定存在不足之处，诚恳欢迎读者不吝指正，以便修订时及时更正。

编　者

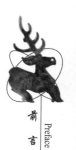

Preface

Language teaching and cultural teaching are inseparable, because language is the carrier of culture. International students studying in China not only need to master basic skills such as listening, speaking, reading and writing in Chinese, but also need to understand traditional cultural knowledge with Chinese characteristics. Only by driving language learning with rich cultural basic knowledge, can the learning task be better completed. At the same time, cultural experience can effectively promote the cultural identity and improve the effect of cultural teaching by providing a real cultural environment and guiding students to experience it in person. It is an important part of the cultivation of foreign students majoring in traditional Chinese medicine to train foreign students in China who major in traditional Chinese medicine and guide them to study the Chinese culture, including the culture of the Central Plains and the traditional Chinese medicine. Therefore, it is imperative to compile teaching materials of traditional Chinese medicine culture that are conducive to "teaching" and "learning".

At present, the cultural teaching of international students in China has problems such as the convergence of teaching contents, the single teaching mode, the lack of experience bases, and the lack of teaching themes, which seriously restrict the cognition and recognition of Chinese culture and traditional Chinese medicine culture for international students in China. In order to solve the above problems, in the process of writing this book, centering on the traditional Chinese medicine culture and being based on the advantages of the Central Plains culture, it highlights four major characteristics: bilingual characteristics, traditional Chinese medicine characteristics, Central Plains characteristics, and Zhongjing characteristics. On the basis of outstanding characteristics, it not only emphasizes the dissemination of the technology, theory and culture of the traditional Chinese medicine, but also puts more emphasis on the cultural characteristics of the Central Plains. This is a solid foundation for compiling a series of teaching materials of the traditional Chinese medicine, which are easy to be understood and disseminated, with great popularity, abundant pictures and bilingual contents.

The book is divided into three chapters, compiled according to the modules of the Central Plains, Traditional Chinese Medicine, and Zhongjing Culture. It is designed for 36 hours of teaching. Teachers can make appropriate adjustments based on the actual teaching situation. At the same time, practical activities and after-school homework are arranged after the teaching content of each chapter. It is suggested that teachers can appropriately increase the experience teaching according to the regional cultural characteristics, increase the proportion of cultural practice teaching, consider the relationship between the theoretical teaching and the practical teaching, and pay attention to the two-way communication between teachers and students in cultural teaching to improve the pertinence and interest of the cultural teaching.

The editors of this book are all front-line teachers who have been engaged in Chinese teaching, cultural teaching, and Chinese medicine teaching for foreign students in China for many years, and have rich teaching experience.

Nevertheless, since the experience teaching of international students in China is still in the exploratory stage, the syllabus and teaching content are significantly different at the school level, and the editorial level is limited.

Editors

C目 录
ontents

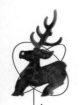

第一章　中原文化体验与实践

第一节　中原文化的形成

　　河南地处黄河中下游，面积跨长江、淮河、黄河、海河四大流域，简称"豫"，"中原"和"中州"也是河南的别称。波澜壮阔的黄河在这里孕育了中华文明，冲积的沃土滋补了此处的生命。早在8 000多年前，河南就出现了农业和定居生活，5 000余年前出现古代城市，4 000年前建立了世界上最早的国家。回望世界古代文明的历程，中华文明作为四大文明中唯一绵延至今的文明，源远流长，而中原地区恰为这一文明保存最为完整的区域。中原文明的发展历程，也是中华文明灿烂辉煌的历史的见证。

　　作为中华文化的母体和主干，中原文化是黄河中下游地区精神文明和物质文化的总称，更是中华文化不可或缺的组成部分乃至其重要源头。中国八大古都中有四座位于河南，即洛阳、开封、安阳和郑州。中原地区以其特殊的地理环境、历史地位和人文精神，在中国漫长的历史长河中长期占据着主流地位。可以说，中原文化在一定程度上成了中国传统文化的代名词。

Chapter Ⅰ Experience and Practice of the Central Plains Culture

Section Ⅰ The Formation of the Central Plains Culture

Henan is located in the middle and lower reaches of the Yellow River, spanning the four major river basins of the Yangtze River, the Huaihe River, the Yellow River and the Haihe River. Fertile soil nourishes life here. Agriculture and settlement life appeared in Henan 8,000 years ago; ancient cities appeared 5,000 years ago, and the world's earliest country was established 4,000 years ago. Looking back at the history of ancient civilizations in the world, the Chinese civilization, as the only civilization among the four major civilizations, has a long history, and the Central Plains is the region with the most complete preservation of this civilization. The development of the Central Plains civilization is also a testimony to the splendid history of the Chinese civilization.

As the mother and backbone of Chinese culture, the Central Plains culture is the general term for the spiritual civilization and material culture in the middle and lower reaches of the Yellow River, and it is an indispensable part of Chinese culture and even its important source. Four of China's eight ancient capitals are located in Henan, namely Luoyang, Kaifeng, Anyang and Zhengzhou. With its special geographical environment, historical status and humanistic spirit, the Central Plains region has long occupied the mainstream position in China's long history. It can be said that the Central Plains culture has become synonymous with traditional Chinese culture to a certain extent.

第二节　中原文化的地位

中原文化是整个中华文明体系的摇篮。这充分体现在史前文明的口头传承或文字记载以来的文明开始。从"盘古开天""女娲造人"等神话故事，到对早期的裴李岗文化、仰韶文化的考古发掘，自成序列，精彩迭呈。夏、商、周三个朝代的文化同样发端于河南，被视为中华文明的根源。作为东方文明标志的儒家、道家、墨家、法家思想，也正是在研究总结三朝文明的基础上而发源于河南的。中国古代政治制度、思想、文字、商业、重大科技发明与中医药的出现，都烙下了不可磨灭的中原文化印记。《易经》《道德经》《伤寒杂病论》以及张衡的浑天仪，都在中国文明乃至世界文明史上占据着举足轻重的地位。

"嵩岳苍苍，河水泱泱"，感召力和辐射力是中原文化的代名词，中原文化具有开放性、包容性的特点，集中体现在：一是影响深远，如中国南方的岭南文化、闽台文化以及客家文化都来源于中原的河洛文化；二是形成风俗，中原文化的一些礼仪习惯经常被拿来作为统一的范本，教育感化民众，并推广到社会及家庭教育的各个环节中；三是传播异域，秦汉时期，中原文化主要通过陆路交通广泛传播，不仅影响了朝鲜、日本的古代文明，而且开辟了起点为洛阳的丝绸之路，而到了北宋时期，航海技术发达，中原文化通过当时最发达的海上交通，远播南亚、非洲各国。

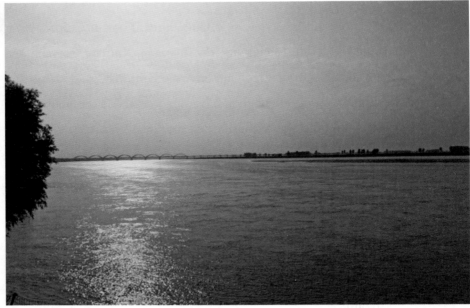

黄河宽景
Wide view of the Yellow River

除此之外，中华文化的核心思想如"大同""和合"，核心价值观如"礼义廉耻、仁爱忠信"，重大民俗活动如婚丧嫁娶、岁时节日，都来源于中原文化及民俗。

Section II The Status of the Central Plains Culture

The Central Plains culture is the cradle of the entire Chinese civilization system. This is fully reflected in the oral inheritance of prehistoric civilization or the beginning of civilization since written records. From the mythological stories of "Pangu created the heaven" and "Nüwa created human", to the archaeological excavations of the early Peiligang culture and Yangshao culture, it has formed a sequence of its own and has been wonderfully repeated. The cultures of the Xia, Shang and Zhou dynasties also originated in Henan and are regarded as the root of Chinese civilization. Confucianism, Taoism, Mohism and Legalism, which are the symbols of eastern civilization, originated in Henan on the basis of studying and summarizing the civilizations of the three dynasties. The emergence of ancient Chinese political system, thought, writing, commerce, major scientific and technological inventions and traditional Chinese medicine has left an indelible mark on the culture of the Central Plains. *The Book of Changes, Tao Te Ching, Treatise on Febrile Diseases and Miscellaneous Diseases*, and Zhang Heng's Armillary Sphere all occupy a pivotal position in the history of Chinese civilization and even the world civilization. "Songyue (Songshan Mountain) is green, (and the) rivers are beautiful." The appeal and radiation are synonymous with the Central Plains culture, which has the characteristics of openness and high inclusiveness. The first characteristic is the far-reaching influence: For example, the Lingnan culture, Fujian-Taiwan culture and Hakka culture in southern China all originate from the Heluo culture in the Central Plains. The second characteristic is the formation of customs: Some etiquette habits in the Central Plains culture are often used as a unified model to educate and influence the people, and promote to the society and family education in each link. The third characteristic is to spread exotic areas: During the Qin and Han dynasties, the Central Plains culture was widely spread mainly through land transportation, which not only affected the ancient civilizations of Korea and Japan, but also opened up a starting point, the Silk Road of Luoyang. In the Northern Song Dynasty, the navigation technology was developed, and the culture of the Central Plains spread to South Asia and Africa through the most developed maritime transportation at that time. In addition, the core ideas of

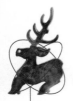

Chinese culture such as "Great Harmony" and "Harmony", core values such as "Propriety, Righteousness, Integrity, Honor, Kindheartedness, Loyalty and Faithfulness", and major folk activities such as weddings, funerals, and festivals all originate from the Central Plains culture and folk customs.

第三节　中原文化的代表符号

一、图腾

在中华文化里,神龙象征着智慧、勇敢、吉祥和尊贵。河南是龙的故乡。中国有记载的创世神——伏羲,在河南周口淮阳一带首次创造了龙形的图腾。相传中国人文始祖之一的黄帝,在统一黄河流域的各个部落后,为了凝聚各部族,也开始使用龙图腾作为新部落的标志。这也是今天中国人被称作"龙的传人"的由来。

6

从在河南出土的文物来看,河南与龙有关的文物不但历史久远,而且最为正统。濮阳蚌龙是中国迄今为止最早的龙形象,距今约6 400年,考古学界称其为"中华第一龙";大型绿松石龙形器在华夏第一王都偃师二里头遗址被发现,距今至少有3 700年,学者将它命名为"中国龙"。这一龙形器的发现,也为中华民族的象征——龙

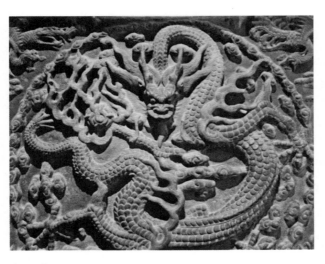

龙图腾
Dragon Totem

找到了最直接、最正宗的根源。中原地区的风俗习惯也有很多与龙相关，如每逢佳节舞龙，农历二月二祭龙王、吃龙须面，端午节赛龙舟等。这些文化除了在中华大地传播承继外，还被远赴海外各地的华人带到了世界各个角落，在世界各国的中国城或唐人街内最具有代表性、最引人注目的装饰就是龙。从中原大地产生并完善的龙形象，目前已成为中华文化的象征、中华民族的象征和促进中华民族大团结的精神支柱。

Section III   Representative Symbols of the Central Plains Culture

|. Totem

In Chinese culture, the dragon symbolizes wisdom, bravery, auspiciousness and dignity. Henan is the hometown of dragons. The recorded god of creation in China, Fuxi, created a dragon-shaped totem for the first time in the area of Huaiyang and Zhoukou in Henan Province. According to legend, Huangdi, one of the ancestors of Chinese humanities, after unifying the tribes in the Yellow River Basin, also began to use the dragon totem as the symbol of the new tribe in order to cohere these tribes. This is also the origin of the Chinese people today who are called "descendants of the dragon".

Judging from the cultural relics unearthed in Henan, the cultural relics related to dragons in Henan not only have a long history, but also are the most orthodox. Puyang Clam Dragon is the earliest dragon image in China, dating back to about 6,400 years ago, which archaeological field called "the first dragon in China"; a large turquoise dragon-shaped vessel was discovered at the Erlitou site of Yanshi, the first capital of China, dating back at least 3,700 years.

Scholars named it "Chinese Dragon". With the discovery of this dragon-shaped utensil, the most direct and authentic source of the dragon and the symbol of the Chinese nation, has been found. There are also many customs and habits in the Central Plains related to dragons, such as dragon dances on festivals, offering sacrifices to the Dragon King on the second day of the second lunar month, eating dragon beard noodles, and dragon boat racing on the Dragon Boat Festival. In addition to spreading and inheriting these cultures in China, they have also been brought to all corners of the world by Chinese who have traveled overseas. In Chinatowns around the world, the most representative and eye-catching decoration is the dragon. The dragon image, which was born and perfected in the Central Plains, has now become a symbol of Chinese culture, a symbol of the Chinese nation, and a spiritual pillar to promote the great unity of the Chinese nation.

实践活动

1. 参观河南开封龙亭公园，寻找"龙"的足迹。

2. 观看舞龙表演，体验中国舞龙文化。

3. 观看或体验赛龙舟活动。

课后作业

1. 谈谈你对中国龙的印象或看法，并讨论问题：中国的龙和你们国家的龙在形象上有什么区别？

2. 临摹一幅中国龙的图画或拍摄带有中国龙图案的照片。

Practice

1. Visit Longting Park in Kaifeng to look for the footprints of the "dragon".

2. Watch the dragon dance performance and experience the Chinese dragon dance culture.

3. Watch or experience dragon boat racing.

Homework

1. Talk about your impressions or views on Chinese dragons, and discuss the question: What is the difference in image between Chinese dragons and your country's dragons?

2. Copy a picture of a Chinese dragon or take a photo with a Chinese dragon pattern.

二、汉字与语言

1. 汉字的起源

相传黄帝时期的仓颉在河南创造发明了文字。据记载，仓颉是黄帝时期负责造字的史官，某天他受到鸟兽足迹的启发，通过仔细观察身边事物的形象，创造出一系列文字。他还经常研究整理先民使用的象形文字符号，并在社会上推广，使文字得以传播。仓颉作为文字的发明者，为人类的交流开辟了新的途径，因此他也在诸多为"汉字"做出贡献的智者中被当作代表和象征。以此形象为仓颉所造出的字体，被称为汉字。他所创的文字有六类大意，也就是汉字的"六书"原则。

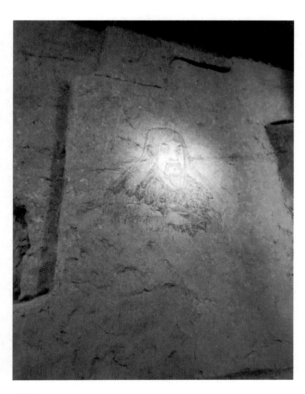

仓颉
Cang Jie

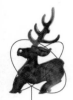

第一类是指象形字，如"日、月"是指象形文字，日满月亏，仿照其形也。

第二类是指代事情的字，如"上、下"是指事情，在上为上，在下为下。

第三类是指会意字，如"武、信"为表会意的文字，止戈为武，人言为信也。

第四类是指形声字，以类为形，配以声。如"江、河"的左边是形，右边是声音。

第五类是指转注字，如"老、考"，以老寿考也。

第六类是指假借字，如"其、我"。数言同字，其发音虽然不一样，意思却相同。

Ⅱ. Chinese Characters and Language

1. The origin of Chinese characters

According to legend, Cang Jie in the Yellow Emperor Period invented characters in Henan. According to records, Cang Jie was the historian who was responsible for coining characters during the Yellow Emperor Period. One day, inspired by the footprints of birds and beasts, he created a series of characters by carefully observing the images of things around him. He also often conducted researches and sorted out the pictographic symbols used by the ancestors, and promoted them in the society, so that the characters could be spread. As the inventor of characters, Cang Jie opened up a new way for human communication, so he was also regarded as a representative and symbol among many wise men who have contributed to "Chinese characters". The font created by Cang Jie with this image is called Chinese characters. The characters he created have six categories, that is, the "Six Categoties of Chinese Characters".

The first category is pictograph, such as "the sun and the moon", which refers to pictographs.

The second category refers to things, such as "being up and down".

The third category refers to the character that is comprehensible. For example, "Wu, Xin" is the character that expresses understanding. " 武 (Wu)" is the synthesis of two characters " 止 " and " 戈 ", meaning the martial arts. People's words are " 信（Xin）." Therefore, to stop the war is the real kung fu.

The fourth category is the phonetic character, categorized by the shape accompanied by the sound. For example, in " 江 *jiang* and 河 *he* (river)", the left side is the shape, and the right side is the sound.

The fifth category refers to the transfer of annotation characters, such as "Lao, Kao", which is based on Lao, shou, Kao.

The sixth category refers to borrowed characters, such as "Qi, Wo". Although the pronunciation is different, the meaning is the same.

2. 甲骨文与现代汉字

甲骨文，是我国最早的汉字形式，又称"契文""甲骨卜辞""殷墟文字"或"龟甲兽骨文"，主要指中国商朝晚期王室用于占卜吉凶，并将占卜之辞和相关的事情契刻在龟甲或兽骨上的文字。商朝时期的文字刻在甲骨上是用来占卜的。随着商朝的衰落和灭亡，文字也进入了一个新的历史时期。

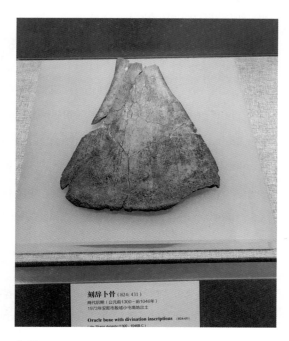

刻辞卜骨（H24: 431）
商代后期（公元前1300—前1046年）
1973年安阳市殷墟小屯南地出土

Oracle bone with divination inscriptions (H24:431)
Late Shang dynasty (1300 - 1046B.C.)

卜骨
Bone

最早发现甲骨文的，是河南安阳小屯村的村民们，他们当时不知道这是古代的遗物，把刻着甲骨文的龟甲兽骨磨成粉末，当作药材使用，因此许多极为有价值的文物被浪费。后来，金石学家王懿荣于光绪二十五年从在药房买来的甲骨上发现了甲骨文。从那之后，当地通过考古发掘及其他途径的探索，已有超过 154 600 件甲骨被出土。

　　此外，河南其余地区乃至陕西、山东等地甲骨文也陆续出现，可追溯到商晚期（约公元前 1300 年）一直至春秋时期。

　　2. Oracle bones and modern Chinese characters

　　Oracle bone inscriptions are the earliest forms of Chinese characters in my country, also known as "Qiwen", "oracle bone inscriptions", "Yinxu inscriptions" or "tortoise shell and animal bone inscriptions" and related things inscribed on tortoise shells or animal bones. The characters of the Shang Dynasty were engraved on oracle bones for divination. With the decline and demise of the Shang Dynasty, writing also entered a new historical period.

　　The villagers of Xiaotun Village in Anyang, Henan Province were the first to discover the oracle bone inscriptions. They did not know that it was an ancient relic. They ground the tortoise shell animal bones engraved with oracle bone inscriptions into powder and used them as medicinal materials. Therefore, many extremely valuable cultural relics were wasted. Later, in the twenty-fifth year of Guangxureign, epigraphist Wang Yirong discovered oracle bone inscriptions on oracle bones bought at a pharmacy. Since then, more than 154,600 oracle bones have been unearthed through archaeological excavations and other means of exploration. In addition, oracle bone inscriptions appeared one after another in the rest of Henan, and even in Shaanxi, Shandong and other places, dating back to the late Shang Dynasty (about 1300 BC) to the Spring and Autumn Period.

　　3. 汉字造字规律与通用印刷

　　河南漯河人许慎于公元 100 年编写了中国首部字典《说文解字》，

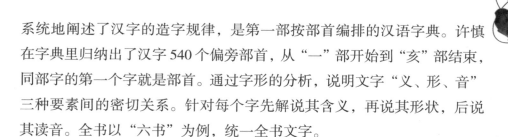

系统地阐述了汉字的造字规律，是第一部按部首编排的汉语字典。许慎在字典里归纳出了汉字 540 个偏旁部首，从"一"部开始到"亥"部结束，同部字的第一个字就是部首。通过字形的分析，说明文字"义、形、音"三种要素间的密切关系。针对每个字先解说其含义，再说其形状，后说其读音。全书以"六书"为例，统一全书文字。

宋体产生于北宋的都城河南开封，是由北宋时期开封的宰相秦桧发明的，因其刻写方便，字体便于识别，广泛流传于后世。印刷术的发明为宋体的产生奠定了基础，宋朝时期文化繁荣，使印刷业有了空前的发展。笔画的粗细变化被宋体体现得淋漓尽致，大部分是横细竖粗，如宋徽宗的瘦金体等。点、捺、钩、撇等笔画有尖端，在报纸、书籍印刷的正文排版中也常被广泛采用。作为中国古代的四大发明之一的活字印刷术也产生于开封。

3. The rules of Chinese character creation and general printing

Xu Shen, a native of Luohe, Henan, wrote China's first dictionary *Shuowen Jie Zi* in 100 AD, which systematically expounded the rules of Chinese character creation. It was the first Chinese dictionary organized according to radicals. Xu Shen summed up 540 radicals of Chinese characters in the dictionary, starting from the "一" part and ending with the "亥" part. The first character of the same part is the radical. The close relationship among three elements, "meaning, shape and sound" is explained through the analysis of the characters. For each character, it first explains meaning, then shape, and its pronunciation. The whole book takes "the six categories of Chinese characters" as an example to unify the entire text.

Born in Kaifeng, Henan, the capital of the Northern Song Dynasty, the Song Typeface was invented by Qin Hui, the prime minister of Kaifeng in the Northern Song Dynasty. The invention of printing has undoubtedly laid the foundation for the emergence of the Song Typeface. The cultural prosperity

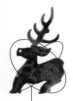
of the Song Dynasty made the printing industry have an unprecedented development.

The degree of thickness changes was vividly reflected in the Song Typeface, and most of them are horizontally thin and vertically thick, such as the Thin Gold Typefaceof during the period of Emperor Huizong of the Song Dynasty. Strokes such as dot, pierce, hook, and skimming are sharp, and are often widely used in the text layout of newspapers, books, and magazines. As one of the four great inventions of ancient China, movable type printing was also produced in Kaifeng.

4. 语言——河南话

汉语中的官话是一直通行于以洛阳为中心的北方广大地区的使用人口最多、分布范围最广泛的方言。中国目前统一使用的普通话就是官话。黄河在河南孕育了中原文化，而中原文化造就了中原官话。

历史上，河南方言常被北方官话区作为统一标准，来规范自己的语汇以及语法系统。追溯至古代，商朝的语言是汉语中原官话的雏形。东周通用全国的语言就是以洛阳话为标准的华夏语。明清时期是河南方言的基本成型期，正如今天的中原官话一样，几千年的融会贯通使近代的河南方言得以生成。

中原文化在河南本土也表现出强大的生命力，最典型的就是常用语"中"。"中"是河南全省通用的一个词，意思相当于普通话的"行、好、可以"。河南人喜欢说"中"的原因：一方面可能与河南地处中原，一贯以中州自居有关；另一方面也体现了河南人说话言简意赅、直爽朴实的特点。

4. Language—Henan dialect

Mandarin in Chinese is the dialect with the largest population and the widest distribution in the vast northern region centered on Luoyang. Mandarin is the standard language in China at present. The Yellow River gave birth to the Central Plains culture in Henan, and the Central Plains culture created the

Central Plains Mandarin.

Historically, Henan dialect was often used as a unified standard by the northern Mandarin area to standardize its own vocabulary and grammar system. Dating back to ancient times, the language of the Shang Dynasty was the prototype of Mandarin Chinese in the Central Plains. The national language in the Eastern Zhou Dynasty was Huaxia Language with Luoyang dialect as the standard. The Ming and Qing dynasties were the basic formative periods of Henan dialect. Just like today's Mandarin in the Central Plains, the modern Henan dialect came into being after thousands of years of integration.

The Central Plains culture also shows strong vitality in Henan itself. " 中 *Zhong*(middle)" is a word commonly used in Henan province, which means "OK" in Mandarin. On the one hand, Henan people like to say "Zhong", which may be related to the fact that Henan is located in the Central Plains and has always regarded itself as Zhongzhou; On the other hand, it also reflects Henan people's concise, straightforward and simple characteristics.

实践活动

1. 参观河南郑州市博物馆，了解中国文字的历史。

2. 研究一下甲骨文，临摹一个汉字的甲骨文形式。

3. 与河南老百姓交谈，感受一下河南方言。

课后作业

1. 通过甲骨文到现代汉字的演变，找一些汉字学习的方法和经验，可以小组讨论，形成一份书面报告。

2. 学习 1 ~ 3 句河南方言并理解其含义。

3. 在你的脑海里，河南省的轮廓是什么形状的？

Practice

1. Visit the Zhengzhou Museum in Henan to learn about the history of

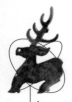

Chinese characters.

2. Study the oracle bone inscriptions and copy the oracle bone inscriptions of a Chinese character.

3. Talk to ordinary people in Henan and experience the Henan dialect.

Homework

1. Through studying the evolution of oracle bone inscriptions to modern Chinese characters, find some methods and experiences of Chinese character learning, and discuss in groups to form a written report.

2. Learn 1 to 3 sentences of Henan dialect and understand their meanings.

3. In your mind, what is the shape of the profile of Henan Province?

三、艺术

1. 文学

中原地区是汉文明的起源地，而中原文学又是中国文学的根源。中国最早的散文总集《尚书》和诗歌《诗经》都出自中原地区。中原辞赋散文在汉代文学史上有着举足轻重的地位，中原文学的基本艺术特征在汉魏时期被确立，并有"汉魏文章半洛阳"之说。魏晋时期，受时代风气的影响，文人的文体与创作观念都发生了较大的变化，中原诞生了建安风骨、正始之音。左思的《三都赋》还使得"洛阳纸贵"的佳话得以流传。与此同时，中原士族向南方迁移，促进了江南文学的繁荣。隋唐时期，中原文学空前繁荣，文学作品数不胜数，并且名家辈出。唐代留名的两千多名作家中，有五分之一被河南人士所占据。唐代三大诗人中杜甫和白居易都来自中原，位居"唐宋八大家"之首的韩愈也来自河南孟州。北宋时期，东京（今开封）作为世界级的繁华都会，勾栏瓦舍遍布，说唱艺术勃兴，极大地促进了宋词和话本小说的产生和兴盛。南宋之后，北方战乱频繁，致使中原文化被迫向南迁移，中原文学才逐渐衰落。即便如此，在元、明、清时期，中原地区仍然不乏李梦阳这样的著名文学家。

经过不断努力，近代中原作家在 19 世纪末被文学界授予了"文学豫军"的称号。

Ⅲ. Art

1.Literature

The Central Plains is the origin of the Han civilization, and the Central Plains literature is the root of Chinese literature. The earliest Chinese prose collection the *Book of History* and the *Book of Poetry* were from the Central Plains. The Central Plains' poetry and prose played an important role in the literature history of the Han Dynasty. The basic artistic characteristics of the Central Plains literature were established in the Han and Wei dynasties, and there was a saying that "Half of the Han and Wei articles came from Luoyang". During the Wei and Jin Dynasties, under the influence of the ethos of the times, the literati's style and creative concept had undergone great changes. Zuo Si's "Ode to the Three Capitals" also made the idiom story of "overwhelming popularity of the work causing the shortage of printing paper in Luoyang" spread. At the same time, the migration of the Central Plains nobility to the south promoted the prosperity of Jiangnan literature. During the Sui and Tang dynasties, the literature of the Central Plains was unprecedentedly prosperous, with numerous literary works and famous scholars. Among more than 2,000 famous writers in the Tang Dynasty, one-fifth of them were occupied by people from Henan. Two of the Three Poets of the Tang Dynasty, Du Fu and Bai Juyi, both came from the Central Plains. Han Yu, who ranked first among the "Eight Great Masters of the Tang and Song dynasties", also came from Mengzhou, Henan. During the Northern Song Dynasty, Dongjing(now Kaifeng), as a world-class prosperous city, was full of theatres , and the art of rap and singing flourished, which greatly promoted the generation and prosperity of Song Poems and vernacular novels. After the Southern Song Dynasty, due to the frequent wars in the north, the culture of the Central Plains was forced to migrate to the south, and the literature of the Central Plains gradually declined. Even so, in the Yuan, Ming and Qing dynasties, there were still many famous writers such as Li Mengyang in the Central Plains. After continuous efforts, the modern Central Plains writers were awarded the title of "Literary Writers of Henan" by the literary circles at the end of the nineteenth century.

2. 音乐

中原音乐文化的体现形式，不仅有中原地区的民乐、民歌以及历史悠久的各种曲艺形式，又有源远流长、保存至今的各种音乐文物和音乐思想。它是中原地区人民生活的真实反映，也是以今河南省为中心的黄河中下游地区的人们创造的一切关于音乐的物质和精神文明的总和。河南省漯河市舞阳县的贾湖遗址出土了被誉为中国第一笛的贾湖骨笛，距今约9 000年至7 700年，是中国目前出土年代最早的乐器实物，至今仍可进行演奏。

中原音乐文化的历史，史书中有葛天氏之乐、神农氏削桐为琴、关于大禹治水的《大夏》歌舞、周王招饮群臣诸侯"呦呦鹿鸣，食野之苹"、商人"恒舞于宫，酣歌于室"。于殷墓出土的三件一组的编磬、两汉魏晋隋唐一承的箫鼓乐队画像砖，唐朝的民间曲子与说唱，以及宋元时期大量的民间音乐形式，都是中原音乐文化的绵延不断的辉煌见证者。

2. Music

The embodiment of the music culture in the Central Plains is not only the folk music, folk songs and various forms of folk art with a long history in the Central Plains, but also various musical cultural relics and music ideas that have a long history and are preserved to this day. It is a true reflection of the life of the people in the Central Plains, and it is also the sum of all the material and spiritual civilizations about music created by the people in the middle and lower reaches of the Yellow River with Henan Province as the center. The Jiahu bone flute, known as the first flute in China, was unearthed at the Jiahu site in Wuyang County, Luohe City, Henan Province. It dates from about 9,000 to 7,700 years ago. It is the earliest real musical instrument unearthed in China, and it can still be played today.

The history of music culture in the Central Plains, the history books include Ge Tian's music, Shennong's cutting tongs for *qin*, the song and dance of "Da Xia" about Dayu's water control, Zhou Wang's invitation to drink his ministers and princes "Mewing and mewing, the deer cry, grazing on wild wormwood", Merchants "dance in the palace and sing in the room". Unearthed in the tomb of Yin—a set of three-piece chimes, one inherited from the Han, Wei, Jin, Sui and Tang Dynasties-the portrait bricks of the Xiao and Drum Band, the folk songs and rap of the Tang Dynasty and the Song Dynasty A large number of folk music forms in the Yuan Dynasty are all glorious witnesses of the continuous and continuous music culture of the Central Plains.

3. 绘画

中原绘画具有悠久历史，最早可追溯至史前新石器时代，如陕县庙底沟出土的花瓣纹陶盆彩绘和汝州阎庄出土的彩陶缸上的鹳鱼石斧图等文物均在这一时期出土，均是史前平面美术遗迹。在中原地区，先秦时期的壁画和漆画作品中，人物和动物的形象描绘已经体现出了生动特点。

中原绘画中，不同的审美取向来自不同时期，晋尚韵、唐尚法、宋尚理、元尚意、明尚趣被体现得淋漓尽致。北宋时期，中原绘画作品已经达到当时全国的巅峰水准，张择端创作的《清明上河图》对于各种形态的几何正确描绘使其负有盛名。

3. Painting

Paintings in the Central Plains have a long history and can be traced back

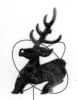

to the prehistoric Neolithic Age, such as the painted pottery pots with petal patterns unearthed in Miaodigou, Shanxian County, and the pictures of storks, fish and stone axes on painted pottery jars unearthed in Yanzhuang, Ruzhou. Unearthed during the period, they were all prehistoric graphic art relics. In the Central Plains, in the frescoes and lacquer paintings during the pre-Qin period, the depiction of figures and animals already showed vivid features. In the paintings of the Central Plains, different aesthetic orientations undoubtedly came from different periods. The preference of the Jin Dynasty for rhyme, the preference of the Tang Dynasty for law, the preference of the Song Dynasty for Neo-Confucianism and the preference of the Yuan Dynasty for artistic conception and the preference of the Ming Dynasty for delight were vividly reflected. During the Northern Song Dynasty, the paintings of the Central Plains had reached the peak in the country at that time. Zhang Zeduan created "Along the River during the Qingming Festival", which was famous for its geometrically correct depiction of various forms.

4. 戏剧、歌曲

夏、商、周的都城都在河南境内，两汉和隋唐时期中国"百戏"活动的中心都在洛阳。

豫剧，起源于河南开封，是中国最大的地方剧种，与京剧、越剧、黄梅戏、评剧并称为中国五大剧种。主要流行于黄河、淮河流域。

豫剧因早期演员用本嗓演唱，起腔与收腔时用假声翻高尾音带"讴"（ōu），又被称为"河南讴"，是在河南梆子的基础上，不断进行守正创新而发展起来的。那为什么将该剧种定名为"豫剧"呢？正是因为河南省的简称是"豫"。其在江苏、山东的部分地区仍被称为梆子戏，在安徽北部地区则被称为梆剧。

豫剧艺术古今兼备，刚柔结合，豁达大方，具有"中和"之美。首先，豫剧唱腔充满激情、雄壮、内敛、激情奔放的阳刚之气，具有强大的情感力量。豫剧音色优美，善于表达人物的内心。此外，豫剧节奏清晰有力，矛盾冲突尖锐，故事有始有终，旋律幽默欢快，不仅适合表演轻松的喜剧，也适合表演帝王将领的盛大场面。豫西戏曲委婉优美，唱腔伤感，非常适合表演悲剧。豫剧一般在关键情节中安排一个大棋盘演唱，演唱流畅、有节奏、富有挑战性。一般来说，发音清晰易懂。

河南曲剧也称"曲子戏"或"高台曲"，有些地区又称之为"南阳曲子"，在中原地区流行。作为河南三大剧种之一的越调，因其伴奏乐器以四胡为主，故又被称作"四股弦"。

歌曲《编花篮》有浓郁的河南韵味，以调式音开头和结尾的音乐形成首尾呼应，调式五度音也以旋律骨干音为特点，偏音的运用充分体现了中原音乐色彩。此曲主要靠运"腔"来体现河南音乐所特有的"语言魅力"。 这首歌曲歌词清新朴实，旋律明朗欢快，饱含"河南元素"，深受人们喜欢。歌词如下：

编，编，编花篮，编个花篮上南山。南山开满红牡丹，朵朵花儿开得艳。银个丹丹嘿银牡丹，银牡丹那个哪哈依呀嗨。

摘，摘，摘牡丹，三朵两朵摘一篮。花儿开得多娇艳，姑娘见了好喜欢，哎嗨哎嗨好喜欢，齐争艳那个哪哈依呀嗨，祖国春色没个边。

4. Drama, Song

The capitals of Xia, Shang and Zhou were all in Henan, and the center of China's "Hundred Opera" activities during the Han and Sui and Tang dynasties were all in Luoyang.

Yu Opera, originated in Kaifeng, Henan Province, is the largest local opera genre in China which is mainly popular in the Yellow River, Huai River Basin. Together with Peking Opera, Shaoxing Opera, Huangmei Opera and Ping Opera, it is one of the five major operas in China.

Yu Opera was developed based on Henan Wooden Clappers with constant innovation and integrity, which is also known as "Henan Ou", as early

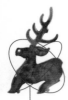

performers sang in their original voice and used a falsetto to raise the end or "ōu" when they started or ended the cavity. Then why is the drama named "Yu Opera"? It is precisely because the abbreviation of Henan Province is "Yu". It is still called Bangzi Opera in some areas of Jiangsu and Shandong, and in northern Anhui it is called Bang Opera.

Yu Opera is both ancient and modern art, combining rigidity and softness, which is open-minded and generous and has the beauty of "neutralization". First of all, the singing of Yu Opera is full of passion, majesty, restraint, and unrestrained masculinity, and has strong emotional power. In addition, Yu Opera has a beautiful tone and is good at expressing the hearts of the characters. Besides, the rhythm of Yu Opera is clear and powerful; the contradictions and conflicts are sharp; the story has a beginning and an end; and the melody is humorous and cheerful. It is not only suitable for performing light comedy, but also for performing grand scenes of emperors and generals. Yu opera in western Henan is euphemistic and beautiful, with a sad voice, which is very suitable for performing tragedy. Yu Opera generally arranges a large chessboard to sing in key plots. The singing is smooth, rhythmic and challenging. Generally speaking, the pronunciation is clear and easy to understand.

Henan Qu Opera is also called "Quzi Opera" or "Gaotai Opera", and in some areas it is also called "Nanyang Quzi", which is popular in the Central Plains. As one of the three major operas in Henan, Yuetiao is also called "Siguxian" because its accompaniment instruments are mainly Sihu.

The song "Weaving Flower Baskets" has a strong Henan charm. The music at the beginning and the end of the modal tone forms the first and last echoes. The modal tone of fifth degree is also characterized by the backbone tone of the melody. The use of partial tone fully reflects the color of the Central Plains

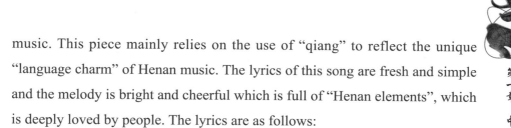

music. This piece mainly relies on the use of "qiang" to reflect the unique "language charm" of Henan music. The lyrics of this song are fresh and simple and the melody is bright and cheerful which is full of "Henan elements", which is deeply loved by people. The lyrics are as follows:

Weave, weave, weave flower baskets, weave a flower basket to Nanshan. Nanshan is full of red peonies, and the flowers are blooming brilliantly. Silver peony. Hey, silver peony, silver peony. Pick, pick, pick peonies, and pick a basket of three or two peonies. The flowers are so beautiful. The girls love when seeing them. Hey hey hey, girls love them. Hey hey hey, the flowers are so beautiful that the spring of the motherland has no bounds.

5. 石刻艺术

石刻艺术是我国古代灿烂文化的一个重要组成部分，在现代中华民族艺术宝库中具有举足轻重的地位，有圆雕、浮雕、刻文记事或塑造形象，内容琳琅满目，一应俱全。

中原到处都是古老的石刻。深邃雄伟的汉代石刻，丰富多彩的碑志铭文，庄严肃穆的陵墓，都诠释着民族气质和时代精神。尤其是栩栩如生的佛像形象，留给人们无尽的艺术享受，展现了古代艺术家的鬼斧神工和非凡的审美情趣。

汉代画像石刻多被用于石室、石阙和陵墓上的装饰性建筑构件。汉代人以刀代笔，以石为纸，采用多种雕刻技法，刻出寓意深远、精美绝伦的历史画卷。郑州、南阳、许昌、商丘和浚县等地是河南汉代画像石刻主要的分布地，画像内容多样，艺术风格各异。其传神的造型，简洁刚健的线条，古拙稚朴的意趣，展现了力量之美、动感之美、气势之美，体现了封建社会兴起时期的蓬勃时代风貌。

5. Stone carving art

Stone carving art is an important part of the splendid ancient culture of our country, and plays a pivotal role in the treasure house of modern Chinese

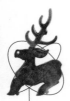

nation art. There are round carvings, relief carvings, engravings to record events or shape images, and the content is dazzling and everything is available.

The Central Plains are full of ancient stone carvings. The profound and majestic stone carvings of the Han Dynasty, the colorful inscriptions on the inscriptions, and the solemn tombs all interpret the national temperament and the spirit of the times. In particular, the lifelike images of Buddha statues leave people with endless artistic enjoyment, showing the fantastic craftsmanship and extraordinary aesthetic taste of ancient artists.

Han Dynasty stone carvings were mostly used for decorative building components on stone chambers, stone towers, and mausoleums. The people of the Han Dynasty used knives as pens, stones as paper, and a variety of carving techniques to engrave historical pictures with far-reaching and exquisite meanings. Zhengzhou, Nanyang, Xuchang, Shangqiu, Hejun County and other places are the main distribution areas of the Han Dynasty portrait stone

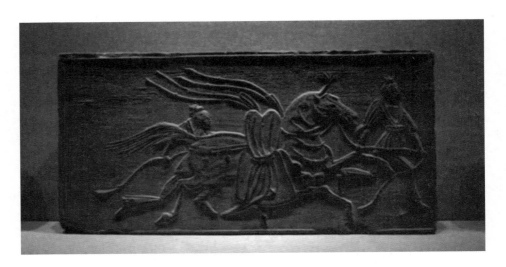

汉代画像石刻

Portrait stone carving in the Han Dynasty

carvings in Henan. The portraits are diverse in content and artistic styles. Its expressive shape, simple and robust lines, and naive interest show the beauty of strength, dynamism, and momentum, and reflect the flourishing style of the times during the rise of feudal society.

实践活动

1. 参观河南豫剧团，了解豫剧的乐器、化装及服饰。

2. 观看豫剧表演，试穿戏服。

3. 学唱豫剧或《编花篮》。

课后作业

1. 谈谈对豫剧的看法。

2. 学唱一首豫剧或歌曲。

Practice

1. Visit the Henan Yu Opera Troupe to learn about the musical instruments, costumes and costumes of Yu Opera.

2. Watch the Yu Opera performance and try on the costumes.

3. Learn to sing Yu Opera or "Weaving Flower Baskets".

Homework

1. Talk about your views on Yu Opera.

2. Learn to sing a Yu Opera or song.

四、中原文物

河南是中国重要的文物大省，历史悠久，文化荟萃，是华夏文明最重要的发源地之一。它绵延着中华民族的血脉和文脉，自先秦流传至今的许多姓氏在这里都可以找到其根源。河南也是中华文明繁荣发展的沃土，数千年的悠长岁月里，河南先民创造出包括青铜器、玉器、陶器等无数巧夺天工又璀璨夺目的文化遗产，无一不展示着河南古代文明的辉煌。"岁月失语，惟石能言"，就让我们走进河南博物院，从出土的文

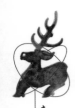

物珍品中感受河南历史文化的独特魅力吧。

河南博物院是民国时期建设而成的国家级博物馆，更是首批中央地方共建国家级博物馆之一。该博物院不仅场地规模较大，而且内部划分明确，具体包括广场、专题陈列馆、临时陈列馆、文物库房、广播室、计算机中心、培训服务楼等。另外，外部还建设有绿化覆盖率40%的园林绿地，因此凭借"馆中园、园中馆"的独特格局吸引人们踊跃前往。其中，主展馆主体建筑的造型形似"戴冠的金字塔"，以元代古观星台为原型。冠部为方斗形，上扬下覆，寓意中原为华夏之源，融汇四方。外部墙面为土黄褐色，寓意华夏文明源于"黄土""黄河"。主馆正面的透明窗与透明采光带，将"黄河之水天上来"的磅礴气势展示得淋漓尽致。整体来看，本建筑群设计强调"中原之气"，线条简洁遒劲，造型别具一格，可谓雄伟壮观、气势恢宏。

17万余件馆藏文物至今被陈列在河南博物院，尤以史前文物、历代陶瓷器、商周青铜器、玉器及石刻最具特色。精品文物数量众多、种类齐全、品位较高、价值连城，是见证中华文明发展轨迹、展示中国历史发展脉络的文化艺术宝库。

Ⅳ. Chinese Cultural Relics

Henan, an important cultural relic province in China, has a long history and rich culture. It is one of the most important birthplaces of Chinese civilization. It stretches the blood and context of the Chinese nation, and many surnames that have been passed down since the pre-Qin period can find their roots here. Henan is a fertile soil for the prosperity and development of Chinese civilization. In the long course of thousands of years, Henan ancestors have created countless ingenious and dazzling cultural heritages including bronze ware, jade ware, pottery and so on, all of which show the splendor of ancient Henan civilization. "Time is aphasia, but stones can speak." Let us walk into the Henan Museum and experience the unique charm of Henan's history and culture from the unearthed cultural relics.

Henan Museum is a national-level museum that was built in the Republic of China era, and also one of the first national-level museums jointly constructed by the central and local governments. In addition to the large-scale site, the museum has a clear internal partition, specifically including a square, thematic exhibition hall, temporary exhibition hall, cultural relic warehouse, broadcasting room, computer center, training service building, etc. Moreover, 40% garden greens have been designed outside, and thus it has attracted a large number of people to visit and stay by virtue of the unique pattern of "garden in museum and museum in garden".

The shape of the major building in the main exhibition hall looks like a "crowned pyramid", which is constructed on the basis of the ancient star observation platform in the Yuan Dynasty. The crown is in the shape of a square bucket, stretching outwards on the top but retracting inwards at the bottom, implying that Central Plains region is the origin of China and integrates various areas around and all over. The external wall is of yellowish-brown color, meaning that Chinese civilization originates from "loess" and "the Yellow River". The

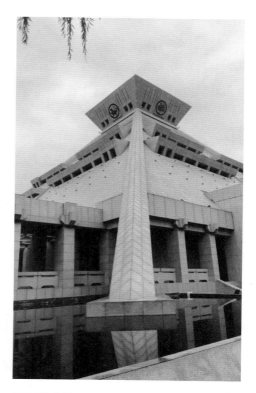

河南博物院
Henan Museum

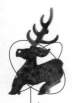

transparent window and daylighting band on the front of the major museum demonstrate the majestic momentum of "the water of the Yellow River coming down from the heaven" incisively and vividly. On the whole, the design of this building complex emphasizes the characteristics of the Central Plains, with simple and powerful lines and a unique modeling, which is really spectacular and magnificent.

More than 170,000 collections of cultural relics have been displayed in the Henan Museum so far, especially prehistoric cultural relics, ceramics of past dynasties, bronzes of Shang and Zhou dynasties, jade and stone carvings. There are a large number of high-quality cultural relics, a complete range, high quality, and invaluable value.

1. 贾湖骨笛

裴李岗文化是目前中原地区发现的时代较早的新石器文化，距今9 000 ~ 7 000 年。河南中部是该类文化的主要分布区，豫北、豫南也有少量发现。磨制石器是其主要生产工具，制作较为精细。骨笛就是这一时期较有代表性的器物。贾湖骨笛距今 8 700 年，用大型禽鸟的肢骨制作而成，上有七孔，管上等分刻画痕迹清晰。它的出土充分反映出先民们高超的音律水平和计算水平，也将中国音乐史向前推进了 3 000 多年，奏响了人类走向文明的最初乐章。

1. Jiahu Bone Flute

The Peiligang culture is an earlier Neolithic culture discovered in the Central Plains, dating back to 9000-7000 years. The ago central part of Henan is the main distribution area of this culture, and a few discoveries have been made in northern and southern Henan. The polished stone implements are the main production tools, and the production is relatively fine. Bone flute is a more representative utensil in this period. The Jiahu bone flute dates back to 8700 years ago. It was made from the limb bones of large birds. Its excavation fully

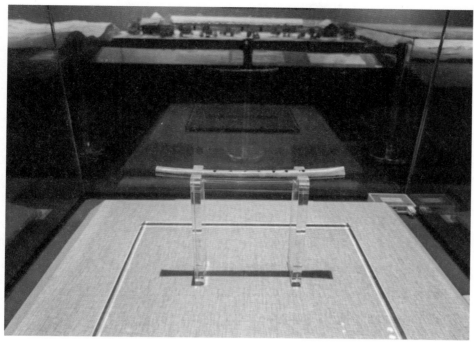

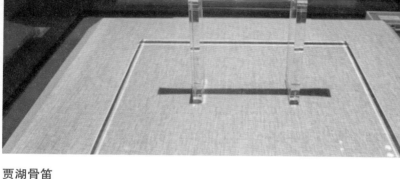

贾湖骨笛
Jiahu Bone Flute

reflects the superb level of rhythm and calculation of the ancestors, and it has also advanced the history of Chinese music for more than 3,000 years, playing the first movement of mankind toward civilization.

2. 杜岭方鼎

夏代晚期都城二里头遗址出土了目前最早的铜鼎实物。在郑州商城及安阳殷墟等商代都邑中开始出现大型成套铜鼎并且装饰兽面纹等图案。

杜岭方鼎是迄今发现的商代早期最大的青铜器之一，鼎口沿外折，两侧沿面上有圆拱形立耳，微微外张，耳的外侧面呈凹槽形，鼎身有八组饕餮纹和乳钉纹规则地分布在四壁的中上部和四周，装饰错落有致，巧妙地创造出富有变化的庄严感，一派王者风范，却又生机勃勃。鼎用于祭祀时炊煮、烹煮、盛放肉食，是先秦时期最具有代表性的立国重器，

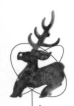

是国家和权力的象征。

2. Du Ling Fang Ding

The earliest bronze tripod was unearthed from the Erlitou site in the late Xia Dynasty. Large sets of bronze tripods began to appear in the Shang Dynasty capitals such as Shangcheng of Zhengzhou and Yinxu of Anyang, decorated with animal face patterns and other patterns.

The Du Ling Fang Ding is one of the largest bronze wares in the early Shang Dynasty discovered so far. Eight groups of taotie patterns and breast nail patterns are regularly distributed in the upper and middle parts of the four walls and around, and the decorations are scattered and ingenious, which subtly creates a sense of solemnity that is rich in changes. It is used for cooking and serving meat in sacrifices. It is the most representative state-building ware in the pre-Qin period and a symbol of state and power.

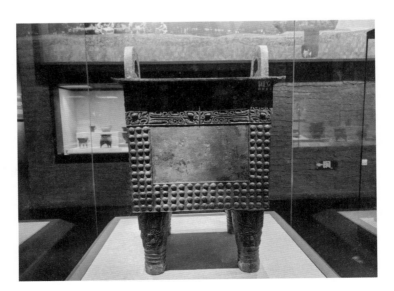

杜岭方鼎
Du Ling Fang Ding

3. 青铜神兽

青铜神兽由三只神兽组成。大神兽为龙首，头顶以六条蛇形龙为角，虎身，龟足，双目圆睁凸起，张口吐舌，獠牙犀利。脊背上有一方座，座上有一神兽也为龙首，口衔一条龙。通身饰动物纹和云纹，满嵌绿松石。此神兽形象诡谲，制作精美，绿松石镶嵌精细，给人极富抽象形式意味的美感，实属罕见之物。

3. Bronze Divine Beast

The bronze divine beast consists of three divine beasts. The big mythical beast has a dragon head, six snake-shaped dragons as horns on the top of its head, a tiger body, tortoise feet, round eyes and protruding eyes, open mouth and tongue, and sharp fangs. There is a seat on the back, and there is a beast on the seat, which is also the head of a dragon, with a dragon in its mouth. Animal and moiré patterns all over the body, all inlaid with turquoise. This mythical beast has a bizarre image, exquisite workmanship, and fine turquoise inlay, giving people a very abstract form of beauty, which is really rare.

31

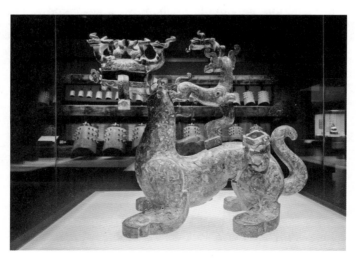

乐器支架 "神兽"
Musical Instrument Stent " Divine Beast"

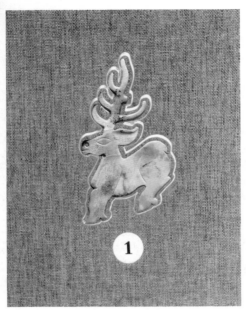

①

鹿形玉佩
Deer-shaped jade pendant

4. 鹿形玉佩

玉鹿是西周动物形玉雕中最具特色的器物，这一时期发现的动物形玉佩多为扁平状，光面无花纹，造型简单，善于以表现局部特征来概括整体外形。这件玉佩在表现鹿的形象时，着力夸大俊美的鹿角，给人一种惟妙惟肖的感觉。

4. Deer-shaped jade pendant

The jade deer is the most distinctive objects in the animal-shaped jade carvings of the Western Zhou Dynasty. Most of the animal-shaped jade pendants found in this period are flat, smooth, and simple in shape without patterns. They are good at expressing local features to summarize the overall shape. When this jade pendant expresses the image of a deer, it focuses on exaggerating the beautiful antlers, giving people a vivid feeling.

实践活动

1. 参观河南博物院。

2. 观看编钟表演。

课后作业

思考问题：为什么河南省电视台的图标是一只大象？

Practice

1. Visit the Henan Museum.

2. Watch the chime show.

Homework

Question to think about: Why is the icon of Henan TV Station an elephant?

第四节　中原名胜古迹

一、嵩山少林寺

1. 地理位置及名称由来

中岳嵩山位于河南省郑州市登封，古称"嵩高山、外方山"，以其地质独特、岩龄古老、构造复杂、保留着形态各异的构造形迹而闻名中外，被称为"世界地质公园"。山上有很多名胜古迹，儒、释、道文化相互交融、蓬勃发展，古建筑群 18 处，其中最具代表性的是少林寺。嵩山少林寺创建于北魏太和十九年（495 年），因其坐落于嵩山腹地少室山茂密丛林之中，故名"少林寺"。

Section Ⅳ　Historical Sites of the Central Plains

Ⅰ. Songshan Shaolin Temple

1. Geographical location and origin of name

Zhongyue Song Mountain is located in Dengfeng, Zhengzhou, Henan Province. It was called "The High Song Mountain or Waifang Mountain" in ancient times. It is famous at home and abroad and is praised as "Global Geopark" for its unique geology, ancient rock age, complex structure, and retention of various structural features. There are many historical sites on the mountain where Confucianism, Buddhism, and Taoism integrate and flourish. There are 18 ancient architectures, and the most representative one is Shaolin Temple. Songshan Shaolin Temple was founded in the 20th year of Taihe in the Northern Wei Dynasty (496). It was named "Shaolin Temple" because it sat in the dense jungle of Shaoshi Mountain in the hinterland of Songshan Mountain.

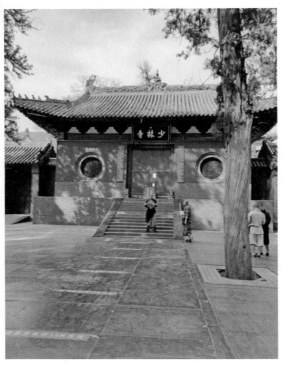

少林寺山门

The Gate of Shaolin Temple

2. 人文景观及其价值

少林寺是中国佛教禅宗的发样地，是世界文化遗产、中国国家重点文物保护单位、国家 AAAAA 级旅游景区，由少林寺常住院、塔林、初祖庵、二祖庵、达摩洞、十方禅院、武术馆以及三皇寨等主要旅游景点组成。少林寺常住院是少林寺的核心，包括山门殿、藏经阁、方丈室、立雪亭等。其中少室晴雪为嵩山八大景观之一，另有达摩"一苇渡江"等传说。

2010 年 8 月 1 日联合国教科文组织第 34 届世界遗产大会审议通过，将包括少林寺常住院、塔林和初祖庵在内的"天地之中"8 处 11 项古建精华列为世界文化遗产，成为中国第 39 处世界遗产。该建筑群历经汉、魏、唐、宋、元、明、清，绵延不绝，构成了一部中国中原地区上下 2 000 多年形象直观的建筑史，是中国时代跨度最长、建筑种类最多、文化内涵最丰富的古代建筑群之一，是中国先民独特宇宙观和审

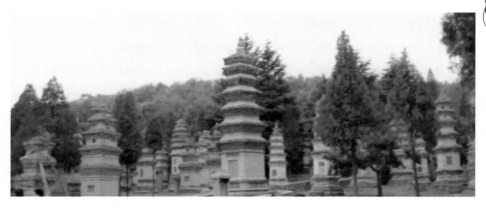

少林寺塔林

The pagodas of Shaolin Temple

美观的真实体现。

2. Humanistic landscape and value

Shaolin Temple is the birthplace of Chinese Zen Buddhism, a world cultural heritage, China's national key cultural relics protection unit, and a national 5A-level scenic area. It is composed of major tourist attractions such as Shaolin Temple, pagodas, Chuzu Temple, Erzu Temple, Bodhidharma Cave, Shifang Buddhist Temple, Wushu(martial art) Hall and Sanhuangzhai(a stockaded village of three emperors). Shaolin Temple's main buildings are its core, including Shanmen Hall, Depositarry of Buddhist Texts, Abbot's Chamber, Lixue Pavilion, etc. Among them, *Shaoshi Qingxue* is one of the eight great landscapes of Songshan Mountain, where there is light reflected on the stone, and there are legends such as "Bodhidharma crossing the river with a reed".

On August 1, 2010, the 34th UNESCO World Heritage Conference reviewed and approved Shaolin Temple and 11 historical buildings in 8 places of "Heaven and Earth" as World Cultural Heritage, becoming China's 39th World Heritage Site. The architectural complex has gone through the Han, Wei, Tang, Song,

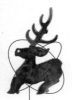

Yuan, Ming, and Qing dynasties, and constitutes a visually intuitive architectural history in the Central Plains of China for 2000 years, ranking as one of the ancient architectural complexes of the longest span in Chinese history, with the most architectural types and the richest cultural connotations. It is the true embodiment of the unique cosmology and aesthetics of the Chinese ancestors.

3. 少林武功

"中国功夫冠天下、天下功夫出少林"，少林寺不仅因其古老神秘的佛教文化名扬天下，更因其精湛实用的少林功夫驰名中外。历史上"十三棍僧救秦王"的典故使少林武功名满天下，少林寺也被封为"天下第一名刹"。少林功夫具有完整的技术和理论体系，以武术技艺和套路为其表现形式，其武功套路高达700种。其因以禅入武，习武修禅，又有"武术禅"之称。至今到寺庙里学习功夫的人还络绎不绝，少林功夫成为世界了解中国的一个重要窗口。

3. Shaolin Kung Fu

"Chinese Kung Fu crowns the world, and the world Kung Fu is based on Shaolin Kung Fu". Shaolin Temple is not only famous for its ancient and mysterious Buddhist culture, but also for its exquisite and practical Shaolin Kung Fu. In history, the story of "Thirteen monks saved the King of Qin" made Shaolin Kung Fu famous for its martial arts, and Shaolin Temple was also named "The first Temple in the world". Shaolin Kung Fu has a complete technical and theoretical system, which takes martial arts skills and routines as its manifestations. There are more than 700 kinds of martial arts routines. It is also known as "martial arts Zen" because it integrates Zen in martial arts and practices martial arts when studying Zen. There is still a constant stream of people who come to the temple to learn Shaolin Kung Fu, and it has also become an important channel for foreigners to learn about China.

4. 文化交流

元、明时期，均有日本国僧人来少林寺修炼佛学，并担任少林寺僧职，与中国僧人结下深厚情谊，至今传为佳话。

自中华人民共和国成立，少林寺与世界各地的文化交流不断提升。外国首脑、政要及国际组织、文化团体等多次参访少林寺，如：英国女王伊丽莎白、南非前总统曼德拉、德国前总理迈克尔等外国元首约见释永信方丈，俄罗斯总统普京、美国前国务卿基辛格、前国际奥委会主席罗格、斯里兰卡前总理贾亚拉特纳，以及国外200余个文化访问团参访少林寺；来自缅甸、泰国、柬埔寨、尼泊尔和斯里兰卡等传统佛教国度的高僧纷纷拜谒；少林寺先后在海外设立数十个少林文化机构，少林寺武僧团先后出访近百个国家与地区，讲经授法、练武修禅，向世界各国传递中华文化的精神内涵和东方价值观；世界各国习练少林功夫及热爱

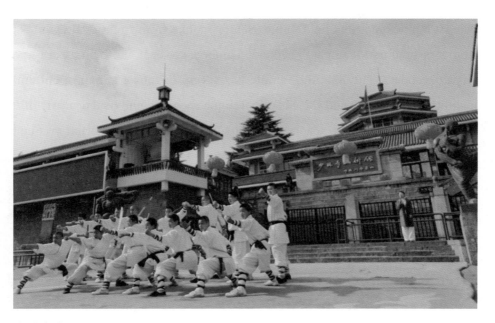

少林武功

Shaolin Kung Fu

少林文化的达数千万人。

4. Cultural exchange

During the Yuan and Ming dynasties, Japanese monks came to Shaolin Temple to learn Buddhism and served in Shaolin Temple. They formed a deep friendship with Chinese monks, which passed down to this day. Since the founding of the People's Republic of China, the cultural exchanges between Shaolin Temple and other parts of the world are constantly improving. Foreign leaders, politicians, international organizations, and cultural groups have visited Shaolin Temple many times. British Queen Elizabeth, South African President Mandela, German Chancellor Michael and other foreign heads of state met with Abbot Shi Yongxin. Russian President Putin, former U.S. Secretary of State Kissinger, International Olympic Committee President Rogge, Sri Lankan Prime Minister Jayaratna, more than 200 foreign cultural delegations visited Shaolin Temple. Senior monks from traditional Buddhist countries such as Myanmar, Thailand, Cambodia, Nepal and Sri Lanka came to pay respects. The Shaolin Temple has set up dozens of Shaolin cultural institutions overseas, and the Shaolin Temple monks have visited nearly 100 countries and regions to teach buddhist scriptures, practice martial arts and Zen, and convey the spiritual connotation of Chinese culture and oriental values to the world. Tens of millions of people around the world practice Shaolin Kung Fu and love Shaolin culture.

实践活动

1. 参观嵩山少林寺，了解体现中国先民独特宇宙观和审美观的建筑。

2. 体验少林功夫，了解中国传统文化。

3. 参观少林药局、少林书局等，体验东方佛学文化。

课后作业

谈一谈对嵩山少林寺的印象（书面或小组讨论）。

Practice

1. Visit Shaolin Temple and learn about the architectures that embody the unique cosmology and aesthetics of the Chinese ancestors.

2. Experience Shaolin Kung Fu and understand traditional Chinese culture.

3. Visit Shaolin Pharmacy, Shaolin Bookstore, etc. to experience Eastern Buddhist culture.

Homework

Talk about your impression of Songshan Shaolin Temple (written or group discussion)

二、洛阳龙门石窟

1. 地理位置及名称由来

龙门石窟位于河南省洛阳市南郊伊河两岸。相传，远古时期龙门山是一个相连的整体，不分东西两山。伊水在龙门山南面汇聚、受阻，

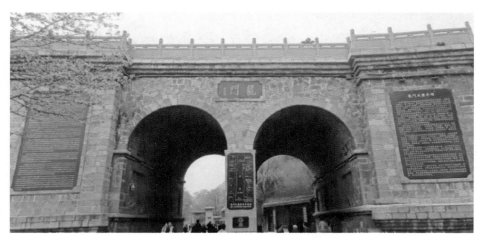

龙门

Longmen

无法向北流出，造成洪水泛滥。因此，大禹把龙门山凿开，分为东西两半（东为香山、西是龙门山），伊水从两山中间向北流出，形似天然门阙，古称伊阙。隋炀帝都洛阳，因伊阙正对皇宫正大门，故而改称"龙门"。

Ⅱ. Luoyang Longmen Grotto

1. Geographical location and origin of name

Luoyang Longmen Grottoes are located on the banks of the Yi River in Luoyang City. Here, the east and west mountains face each other (Xiangshan Mountain on the east and Longmen Mountain on the west). The Yi River flows in the middle and resembles a natural gate, so it was called Yi River Gate in ancient times and also known as Longmen.

2. 人文景观及其价值

洛阳龙门石窟所在的岩体石质优良，宜于雕刻，所以古人选择此处开凿石窟。自北魏孝文帝以来，历经东魏、西魏、北齐、隋、唐、五代、宋等朝代连续大规模营造，从而在这里形成了南北长达1千米、具有

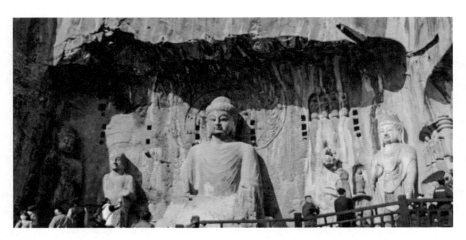

卢舍那大佛
Dalushenaxiang Buddha

2 000余座窟龛和10万余尊造像的石窟遗存。

龙门石窟景区由西山石窟、东山石窟、香山寺和白园四个景点组成。代表洞窟有古阳洞、宾阳中洞、莲花洞、大卢舍那像龛、潜溪寺、敬善寺、万佛洞、惠简洞等。大卢舍那像龛，是武则天根据自己的容貌仪态雕刻的，通高17.14米，头高4米，耳朵长达1.9米，

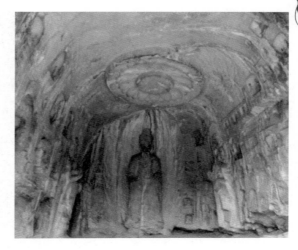

莲花洞
Lotus Grotto

以神秘微笑著称，被国外游客誉为"东方蒙娜丽莎""世界最美雕像"。

莲花洞，因窟顶雕有一朵高浮雕的大莲花而得名，人民大会堂的莲花顶就是依据此莲花设计而成的。莲花周围的飞天体态轻盈，细腰长裙，姿态自如。正壁造一佛二弟子二菩萨，主像为释迦牟尼立像。最小的佛像，仅有2厘米高，生动细致，栩栩如生。

药方洞，刻有140个药方，反映了我国古代医学的成就。把一些药方刻在石碑上或洞窟中，这是古代医学成就传之后世的一个重要方法。

洛阳龙门石窟规模宏大，气势磅礴，延续时间长，跨越朝代多，它保留着大量的宗教、美术、书法、音乐、服饰、医药、建筑和中外交通等方面的实物史料和文字资料，从不同侧面反映了中国古代政治、经济、宗教、文化、艺术等许多领域的发展变化，对中国石窟艺术的创新与发展做出了重大贡献。窟内造像雕刻精湛，内容题材丰富，不仅是中国石刻艺术宝库之一，也被誉为世界最伟大的古典艺术宝库之一。

洛阳龙门石窟为国家AAAAA级旅游景区。2000年11月，联合国教科文组织将龙门石窟列入《世界遗产名录》。

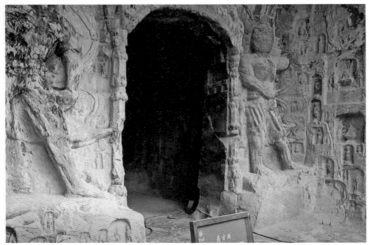

药方洞

Prescription Grotto

实践活动

1. 参观洛阳龙门石窟，体验中国石窟碑刻书法艺术的精华。

2. 关注药方洞，了解中国古代医学传世的方法。

课后作业

讨论中国古代医学传世的其他方法。

2. Cultural landscape and value

Because the rock mass in which the Longmen Grottoes is located is of good quality and suitable for carving, the ancients chose to excavate the grottoes here. The Longmen Grottoes in Luoyang were excavated during the reign of Emperor Xiaowen in the Northern Wei Dynasty, and were successively built on a large scale during the Eastern Wei, Western Wei, Northern Qi, Sui, Tang, Five Dynasties, Song and other dynasties, thus forming the north-south one-kilometer-long cave with more than two thousand niches and the cave with more than 100,000 statues.

Longmen Grottoes consists of four scenic spots: Xishan Grottoes, Dongshan Grottoes, Xiangshan Temple and White Garden. The representative grottoes are Guyang Grotto, Binyangzhong Grotto, Lotus Grotto, Dalushenaxiang Shrine, Qianxi Temple, Jingshan Temple, Wanfo Grotto, Huijian Grotto and so on.

The Dalushenaxiang Shrine is carved by Empress Wu Zetian according to her appearance and posture. It is 17.14 meters high, with the head of 4 meters high and ears of 1.9 meters long. It is known for its mysterious smile and is known as the "Oriental Mona Lisa" and "the most beautiful statue in the world" by foreign tourists.

Lotus Grotto is so named because the top of the cave is carved with a large lotus in high relief. The lotus roof of the Great Hall of the People is based on this lotus design. The flying apsaras around the lotus is light, with thin waist, long skirt and free posture. There are one Buddha, two disciples and two Bodhisattvas in the front, and the main image is Sakyamuni. The smallest Buddha statue is only 2 centimeters high, which is vivid, detailed and lifelike.

The Prescription Grotto is engraved with 140 prescriptions, reflecting the achievements of ancient Chinese medicine. Engraving some prescriptions on stone tablets or caves is an important method for passing on the achievements of ancient medicine to later generations.

The Longmen Grottoes are large in scale and majestic, lasting for a long time and spanning many dynasties. It retains a large number of historical materials and literal data on religion, art, calligraphy, music, clothing, medicine, architecture, and Chinese and international transportation. It reflects the development and changes of ancient Chinese politics, economy, religion, culture, art and many other fields from different aspects, and has made a great contribution to the innovation and development of Chinese grotto art. With

43

exquisite carving and rich subject matter, Longmen Grottoes is not only one of the treasure houses of Chinese stone carving art, but also known as one of the greatest classical art treasures in the world.

As one of nationdl 5A-level scenic areas, in November 2000, UNESCO included the Longmen Grottoes in the "World Heritage List".

Practice

1. Visit the Longmen Grottoes in Luoyang and experience the essence of the art of calligraphy in Chinese stone inscriptions.

2. Observe the medicine cave and understand the methods of ancient medicine passed down from generation to generation.

Homework

Discuss other methods of ancient Chinese medicine inheritance.

三、安阳殷墟与太行大峡谷

1. 殷墟

（1）地理位置及名称由来

殷墟位于河南省安阳市殷都区，横跨洹河南北两岸。大约在公元前

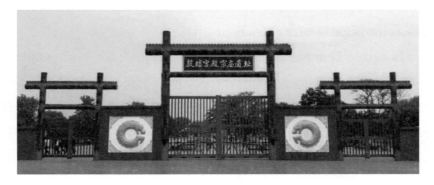

殷墟
Yin Ruins

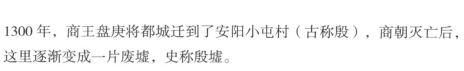

1300 年，商王盘庚将都城迁到了安阳小屯村（古称殷），商朝灭亡后，这里逐渐变成一片废墟，史称殷墟。

（2）人文景观及其价值

殷墟因其出土大量的甲骨文和青铜器而驰名中外，也是中国历史上第一个有文献可考并为甲骨文和考古发掘所证实的古代都城遗址，主要由宫殿宗庙遗址、王陵遗址、后冈遗址和洹北商城遗址等部分组成，是世界文化遗产、国家 AAAAA 级旅游景区、中国考古学的诞生地，也是集考古、园林、古建、旅游为一体的胜地。

殷墟宫殿宗庙遗址内有殷墟车马坑、妇好墓等。妇好墓以墓葬保存完好，墓主人身份明确，出土的随葬品丰富等条件震惊了中外史学界。

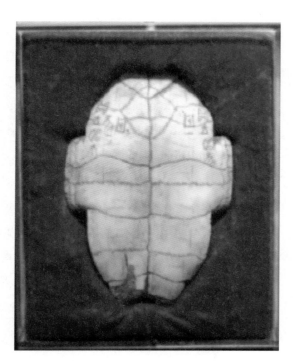

甲骨文
Oracle Bone Inscriptions

殷墟出土了数量众多、制作精美的青铜器、玉器、石器和陶器。青铜器种类繁多，器形厚重，纹饰繁缛，铸造工艺高超，达到了前所未有的水平。其中，司母戊大鼎最负盛名，大鼎高达 133 厘米，器口长 79.2 厘米，重量达 875 千克，是至今世界上发现的最大的青铜器。此鼎造型庞大雄浑，纹饰精美细腻，是古代科技与艺术、雕塑与绘画的完美结合，是中国青铜器文化中的瑰宝。

46

Ⅲ. Anyang Yin Ruins and Taihang Grand Canyon

1. Yin Ruins

(1) Geographical location and origin of the name

Yin Ruins is located in Yindu District, Anyang City, Henan Province, and straddles the Huanhe River. Around 1300 BC, Pan Geng, king of the Shang Dynasty, moved the capital to Xiaotun Village (ancient name Yin) in Anyang. After the collapse of the Shang Dynasty, the place gradually became a ruin, known as Yin Ruins in history.

(2) Cultural landscape and its value

Yin Ruins is famous at home and abroad for its large number of unearthed oracle bone inscriptions and bronzes, which is also the first ancient capital site in Chinese history that was documented and confirmed by oracle bone inscriptions and archaeological excavations. The Yin Ruins is composed of Palace Ancestral Temple relic, Emperor's Tomb, Hougang relic and Huangbei Shangcheng relic, which is world cultural heritage, one of national 5A-level scenic areas, the birthplace of Chinese archaeology, and also a scenic spot integrating archaeology, gardens, ancient architectures, and tourism.

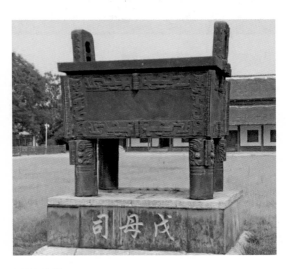

司母戊鼎
Simuwu Ding

There are chariot pit and Fuhao tomb in the relics of Yin Ruins palace and ancestral temple. Fuhao tomb shocks

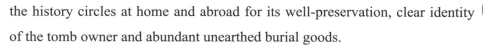

the history circles at home and abroad for its well-preservation, clear identity of the tomb owner and abundant unearthed burial goods.

A large number of exquisitely made bronzes, jades, stone tools and earthenware were unearthed from Yin Ruins. There are many types of bronze wares in Yin Ruins, with heavy shapes, complicated decorations, and superb casting craftsmanship, reaching an unprecedented level. Among them, the Simuwu Ding is the most prestigious, with a height of 133 cm, a mouth length of 79.2 cm, and a weight of 875 kg. It is the largest bronze ware ever found in the world. It is huge and powerful with exquisite and delicate decorations. It is a perfect combination of ancient technology and art, sculpture and painting, a gem of Chinese bronze culture.

2. 太行大峡谷

太行大峡谷位于河南省安阳市林州市石板岩乡境内，南北长50千米，东西宽1.5千米，最高海拔1739米，相对高差1000米以上。峡谷内断崖高起、峰峦叠嶂、怪石峥嵘、流瀑挂壁，姿态万千，是"北雄风光"的典型代表。

太行大峡谷是国家AAAAA级景区，景区总面积89平方千米，自然生态保持良好，植被覆盖率超过90%，有天然氧吧之美誉；其旅游资源丰富，既有儒释道历史文化内涵，又有探险、攀岩、休闲、养生等多种旅游功能。景区主要包括百里画廊太行天路、三九严寒桃花开的"桃花谷"、三伏酷暑水结冰的"太极冰山"，还有太行之魂"王相岩"、潭深谷幽"仙霞谷"等景观，以及亚洲第一、世界一流的国际滑翔基地等。峡谷内民宅就地取材，石街、石院、石墙、石柱、石梯、石楼与大自然浑然一体，古色古香，令人寻味，是观光、绘画、写生的好去处。

太行大峡谷先后获国家森林公园、国家地质公园、中国最美十大峡谷、国家AAAAA级景区、中国攀岩基地等荣誉称号。

2. Taihang Grand Canyon

Taihang Grand Canyon is located in Shibanyan Town, Linzhou, Anyang City, Henan Province. It is 50 kilometers long from north to south, 1.5 kilometers wide from east to west, with an altitude of 800-1739 meters and a relative elevation difference of more than 1,000 meters. The cliffs in the territory are high. The peaks are sturdy. The platform walls are staggered. The waterfalls flow in four directions. The peaks, mountains, platforms, walls, gorges, waterfalls, ridges and springs show various forms, which are a typical representative of "the magnificent scenery in north China". Taihang Grand Canyon is one of national 5A-level scenic areas, with a total area of 89 square kilometers. The scenic area is densely forested, the natural ecology is well

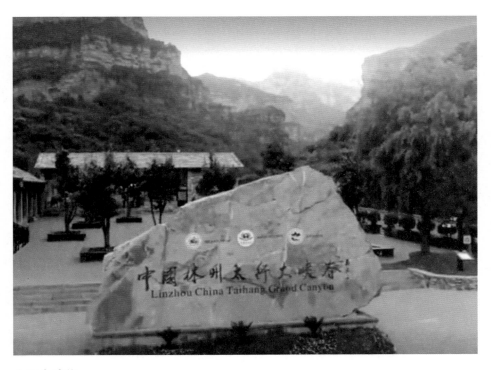

太行大峡谷
Taihang Grand Canyon

maintained, and has the reputation of a natural oxygen bar. Taihang Grand Canyon is rich in tourism resources, which has the historical and cultural connotation of Confucianism, Buddhism and Taoism, as well as a variety of tourism functions such as exploration, rock climbing, leisure and health preservation, including Hundred-mile Gallery—Taihang Road to Heaven, the "Peach Blossom Valley" where peach blossoms bloom in the severe cold winter, the "Taiji Iceberg" where water even gets frozen in hot summer. There are also "Wang Xiang Rock", the soul of Taihang, and "Xianxia Valley" with a deep pond and tranquil valley as well as the first Asian and the world's first-class international gliding base.

The residences in the gorge are made of local materials. The stone streets, stone courtyards, stone walls, stone pillars, stone stairs, and stone buildings are integrated with nature in an antique and intriguing way, which is a good place for sightseeing, painting, sketching and gliding.

Taihang Grand Canyon has won the honorary titles of National Forest Park, National Geological Park, China's ten most beautiful Grand Canyon, National 5A-Level Scenic Area, China rock Climbing Base and so on.

实践活动

1. 参观河南安阳殷墟，探寻中国文字的形成。

2. 参观太行大峡谷，体验中国人文、自然景观。

课后作业

我印象中的中国文字。

Practice

1. Visit the Yin Ruins of Anyang, Henan to explore the formation of Chinese characters.

2. Visit the Taihang Grand Canyon and experience Chinese humanities and

natural landscapes.

Homework

Chinese characters in your impression.

四、开封清明上河园

清明上河园位于河南省开封市龙亭湖西岸，是以北宋张择端的名画《清明上河图》为蓝本，1：1复原再现的大型宋代历史文化主题公园。用巧妙的创意把历史活化，令人有"一朝步入画卷，一日梦回千年"的穿越感，让时光倒流回宋朝，定格在北宋都城（东京）政通人和的政治清明，农业、印刷业、造纸业、丝织业、制瓷业等各行各业重大发展的繁荣景观。行走在城门楼、虹桥、街景、店铺、佛云阁、双宣殿、码头、船坊之间，入目之处皆是北宋的汴绣、服饰、音乐、官瓷、木版年画、曲艺、杂耍、斗鸡、水上百嬉、精美小吃等皇家文化及民间风俗，耳熟能详的包青天、杨家将、梁山好汉、七侠五义等脍炙人口的历史故事都在这里逆着时光上演。体现了主题文化公园集历史文化旅游、民俗风情旅游、休闲度假旅游、趣味娱乐旅游和生态环境旅游于一体的观赏性、知识性、娱乐性、参与性和情趣性等特点。

大型水上实景演出《大宋·东京梦华》，将九阕经典宋词和古画《清明上河图》串联起来，运用高科技手段把宋代的音乐、舞蹈、服饰等融于一体，演绎出了大宋王朝的辉煌，成为展示宋文化魅力和夜游开封的重要载体。

清明上河园占地 0.4 平方千米多，是中原地区最大的仿宋古建筑群，国家 AAAAA 级旅游景区和中国非物质文化遗产展演基地，整个景区展现出一种返璞归真，回归自然的古风与神韵，充分体现了人与自然的和谐统一。

Ⅳ. The Millennium City Park in Kaifeng

The Millennium City Park is located on the west bank of Longting Lake in

来华留学生中原中医药文化体验双语教程

A Chinese-English Course on Traditional Chinese Medicine for Foreign Students in China

Kaifeng City. It is a large-scale Song Dynasty historical and cultural theme park based on the 1:1 restoration and reproduction of the famous Northern Song painter Zhang Zeduan's masterpiece "Along the River during Qingming Festival", which makes people feel like "stepping into the picture in one day, dreaming back to the millennium in one day" and revitalize the history to the Song Dynasty. The Millennium City Park has used great creativity to show the political cleanliness of the Northern Song Dynasty capital (Dongjing), and the prosperous scenes of agriculture, printing, papermaking, silk weaving, porcelain and other industries. Walking in the gate building, Hongqiao, street view, shops, Buddha Cloud pavilion, Shuangxuan Hall, dock, boat lane, we can see Bian embroidery, clothing, music, official porcelain, woodblock New Year pictures, folk art, acrobatic, chicken fighting, water play, exquisite snacks

清明上河园
The Millennium City Park

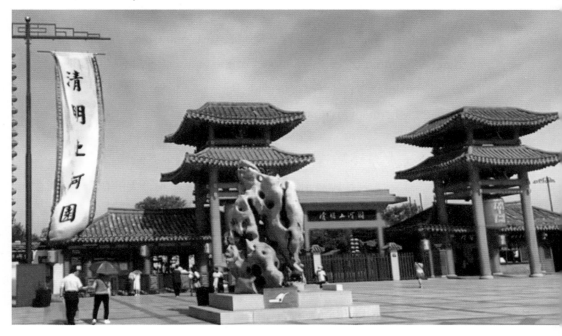

and other royal culture and folk customs of the Northern Song Dynasty. Well-known historical stories such as "Bao Qingtian", "Generals of the Yang family", "Heroes of Liangshan", and "Seven Heroes and Five Gallants" are staged here against the time. The Millennium City Park, as a theme culture park embodies the characteristics of appreciation, knowledge, entertainment, participation and interest of historical and cultural tourism, folk customs tourism, leisure tourism, fun entertainment tourism and ecological environment tourism in one.

There is a large-scale live-action performance "The Great Song Dynasty—Dongjing Dream", which connects the classic Song poems of the Jiuque with the ancient painting "Along the River during Qingming Festival". Using high-tech means to present the splendid Song Dynasty by integrating Song Dynasty music, dance, costumes, etc., this performance has become an important carrier to show the charming culture of the Song Dynasty and night tour of Kaifeng.

The Millennium City Park covers an area of more than 600 acres, and forms the largest group of ancient Song-like buildings in the Central Plains. It is among the first batch of National 5A-Level Scenic Areas and China's intangible cultural heritage exhibition bases. As a model of the national civilized scenic area, the entire area exhibits an ancient style and charm of returning to nature, which fully embodies the harmonious unity of man and nature.

实践活动

1. 参观河南开封清明上河园，体会北宋的繁荣景象。

2. 品尝小吃，体验中国美食文化。

课后作业

根据参观体验，画一幅图画展示"清明上河园"景观。

Practice

1. Visit the Millennium City Park in Kaifeng, Henan, and experience the

prosperity of the Northern Song Dynasty.

2. Taste snacks and experience Chinese food culture.

Homework

Based on the visit experience, draw a picture to show the landscape of the Millennium City Park.

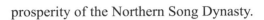

第五节 中原传统工艺

一、洛阳唐三彩

唐三彩主要是指唐代墓葬出土的低温烧造彩色陶瓷制品，造型多变，因为加入铜、铁、钴等元素，在 800℃ 左右的窑温下釉色呈现出绿、赭、蓝三色，故而得名"唐三彩"。但实际上唐三彩远不止这三种釉色，还有白色、绿色、浅蓝、深蓝、黄色、褐色等。

唐三彩主要发现于洛阳和西安两地，但因为发现于洛阳的唐三彩数量较多且时间最早，因此很多人称之为"洛阳唐三彩"。

唐三彩出现于唐高宗时（7 世纪下半叶），盛行于开元年间（8 世纪上半叶），此后渐渐消失。这是因为初盛唐时期社会安定，官民生活富庶，厚葬之风盛行，唐三彩几乎成为达官贵人随葬品中不可或缺之物。

作为冥器，唐三彩被用来模仿复制墓主人生前生活的世界，因此唐三彩器物造型丰富多样，既有日常使用的生活用品，如瓶、壶、罐、钵、杯、盘、盂、烛台、砚台、枕头等，也有建筑以及交通工具模型，如亭台楼榭、仿木箱柜、住房、仓库、牛车、马车等，还有各种俑类，如贵妇、达官、男女侍从、武士、天王、胡人及马、骆驼、猪、羊、鸡、狗等。

在各种造型的唐三彩艺术品中，骆驼与胡人形象最令人印象深刻。唐代中国与世界各国文化经济往来频繁，长安城内常可见到身着胡服、

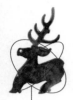

金发碧眼的胡人和外国商队运送货物的骆驼，这是属于大唐的独特风景。唐三彩陶瓷作为人们现世生活的浓缩再现，胡人和骆驼形象自然必不可少。

唐三彩作为广受欢迎的艺术品，也随着胡商经"丝绸之路"远销多个国家。至今，唐三彩不仅发现于中国境内，在印度、日本、朝鲜、伊朗、伊拉克、埃及、意大利等十多个国家也发现有唐三彩。8世纪日本工匠模仿唐三彩，制作出"奈良三彩"，新罗工匠也仿制出"新罗三彩"；9世纪到11世纪，波斯工匠也仿制出"波斯三彩"。

Section Ⅴ　Traditional Crafts of the Central Plains

Ⅰ. Tri-colored Glazed Pottery of the Tang Dynasty in Luoyang

Tang Sancai, also known as Tri-colored Glazed Pottery of the Tang Dynasty mainly refers to the colored ceramic products in low-temperature firing unearthed from the tombs of the Tang Dynasty. The shapes of those art crafts are various. Because of the addition of copper, iron, cobalt and other elements, the glaze color presents green, ochre and blue at the kiln temperature of about 800 degrees, so it is named "Tri-colored Glazed Pottery of the Tang Dynasty". But in fact, there are more than three kinds of glaze colors, including white, green, light blue, dark blue, yellow, brown and so on. The Tri-colored Glazed Pottery was mainly found in Luoyang and Xi'an, but many people called it "Luoyang Tri-colored Glazed Pottery of the Tang Dynasty" because of the large number of tri-colored glazed pottery discovered in Luoyang and the earliest time.

Tri-colored Glazed Pottery of the Tang Dynasty appeared in Gaozong's reign of the Tang Dynasty (the second half of the 7th century), prevailed in Kaiyuan Period (the first half of the 8th century), and then gradually disappeared. This is because in the early Tang Dynasty, the society was stable and officials and people lived a prosperous life, which brought the prevalence of elaborate funeral. As part of the funeral goods, the Tri-colored Glazed Pottery almost was indispensable for high officials and noble lords.

As burial objects, Tri-colored Glazed Pottery of the Tang Dynasty was to imitate life which the tomb owners lived. Therefore, it has various shapes, including daily necessities, such as bottles, pots, cups, plates, bowls, candlesticks, ink stones, pillows, etc. There are also models of buildings and carriages, such as pavilions, wooden cabinets, houses, warehouses, ox carts, carriages, etc. Still, there are figurines, such as ladies, dignitaries, waiters, warriors, heaven kings, the foreign people, horses, camels, pigs, sheep, chickens and dogs, etc.

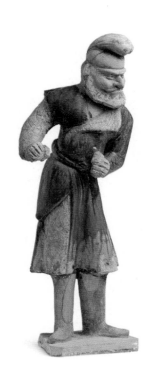

In all kinds of Tri-colored Glazed Pottery of the Tang Dynasty, camels and the foreign people are the most impressive. During the Tang Dynasty, China had frequent cultural and economic exchanges with other countries in the world. In Chang'an City, present city of Xi'an, people

55

三彩胡俑　唐　中国国家博物馆藏

The tri-colored figurines of Hu people from the Tang Dynasty. Collected in the National Museum of China

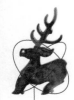

often saw the traders from the west Asia in exotic clothes, with golden hair and blue eyes, and camels used by foreign caravans to carry goods. This is a scene which exclusively belonged to the Tang Dynasty. So, as a concentrated recreation of people's life, the images of the foreign people and camels are very common. As a popular work of art, Tri-colored Glazed Pottery of the Tang Dynasty has also been exported to many countries along with the "Silk Road" by foreign businessmen. So far, Tri-colored Glazed Pottery of the Tang Dynasty has also been found in India, Japan, North Korea, Iran, Iraq, Egypt and Italy. In the 18th century, Japanese craftsmen created Tri-colored Glazed Pottery of Nara based on Tri-colored Glazed Pottery of the Tang Dynasty. Silla craftsmen also imitated the Silla Tri-colored Glazed Pottery. From the 9th century to the 11th century, Persian craftsmen also imitated and produced the "Persian Tri-colored Glazed Pottery".

参考文献

中国硅酸盐学会编. 中国陶瓷史. 文物出版社，1982.

实践活动

1. 参观故宫博物馆陶瓷馆。

2. 参观洛阳博物馆。

课后作业

1. 中国为什么叫 China？

2. 谈一谈"丝绸之路"。

Reference:

1. *History of Chinese Ceramics*, edited by China Silicate Society, Cultural Relics Publishing House, 1982.

2. *Resource Library of Hundreds of Crafts*, Suzhou Arts and Crafts Vocational and Technical College.

Activities

1. Visit the Ceramic Museum of the Forbidden City Museum

2. Visit the Luoyang Museum

Homework

1. Why China is called China?

2. Talk something about the "Silk Road".

二、禹州钧瓷

钧瓷是中国宋元时期北方瓷，出产于河南禹县的钧窑。钧窑，乃宋五大名窑之一，因禹县古属钧州，故名钧窑，其所产瓷器也称钧瓷。宋代钧窑首创釉中加入适量铜，烧成玫瑰紫、海棠红等紫红色釉，色彩艳丽如晚霞。

在此之前，中国陶瓷制品未有如此艳丽的色泽，因此钧瓷被当时的人们视为珍宝。民间自古就有"黄金有价钧无价""家有万贯，不如钧瓷一片"的说法。至北宋后期，钧窑专贡皇室，为宫廷烧制各式花盆与盆托，以供帝王后妃珍养奇花异草。

钧瓷传统造型以盘、钵、碗、炉、花盆等器皿为主，追求端庄大气、质朴自然的艺术风格。钧瓷色彩之多不胜枚举，最知名的有玫瑰红、海棠红、胭脂红、鸡血红、朱砂红、茄色紫、葡萄紫、鹦哥绿、葱茏青、梅子青、天青等。相传以胭脂红、葱茏青和墨色最为难得之佳品。时至今日，游客可以看到更多多姿多彩的钧瓷艺术品，造访位于河南小镇神垕的钧窑旧址，领略千年钧瓷之美。

‖. Jun Porcelain at Yu County

Jun porcelain is the northern porcelain of the Song and Yuan dynasties in China. It was produced in Jun kiln in Yu County, Henan Province. Jun kiln is one of the five most famous kilns in the Song Dynasty. Because Yu County

58

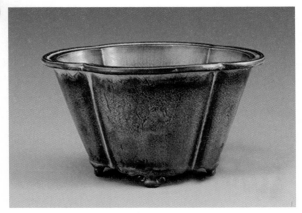

宋 钧窑玫瑰紫釉海棠式花盆

Jun Kiln Rose Purple Glaze Begonia Flower Pot from the Song Dynasty. Collected in the National Museum of China

belonged to Junzhou in ancient world, it was named Jun kiln. Its porcelain is also called Jun porcelain. For the first time, the craftsman created works of art with purplish red glaze of rose purple and begonia red which are colorful as sunset glow by adding appropriate amount of copper.

Before Jun Porcelain was invented, Chinese people never saw porcelains with such gorgeous color, so, they treasured Jun Porcelain. Since that time, a common saying has gons like this, "The gold is valuable, but Jun porcelain is priceless" and "One piece of Jun porcelain is better than a great fortune". In the late Northern Song Dynasty, Jun kilns were special tributes for the royal family, serving all type of flowerpots and pot holders for the imperial concubines to keep rare flowers and plants. The traditional modelings of Jun porcelain are mainly plate, bowl, stove, flowerpot and other utensils, with dignified, simple and natural artistic style. There are many colors of Jun porcelain, the most famous of which are rose red, begonia red, rouge red, chicken blood red, cinnabar red, eggplant purple, grape purple, parrot green, verdant green, plum green, azure, etc. It is said that the rouge, verdant green and ink are the best. Today, visitors can see more colorful Jun porcelain works of art, visit the former site of Jun kiln in Shenhou, a small town in Henan, and enjoy the beauty of Jun porcelain of thousands of years.

参考文献

中国硅酸盐学会编 . 中国陶瓷史 . 文物出版社， 1982.

实践活动

1. 参观神垕古镇钧窑旧址。

2. 参观河南省博物院。

课后作业

谈一谈你对中国历史的了解。

Reference

History of Chinese Ceramics, edited by China Silicate Society, Cultural Relics Publishing House, 1982.

Activities

1. Visit the former site of Jun Kiln at Shenhou, Henan.

2. Visit the Henan Museum

Homework

Talk about everything you know on Chinese history.

三、 朱仙镇年画

年画是中国版画的一种，始于古代的"门神画"，是中国民间艺术之一，常用于春节装饰，含有祝福新年、吉祥喜庆之意。传统民间年画多用木版水印制作，开封朱仙镇、天津杨柳青及苏州桃花坞是中国年画三大中心。

作为中国木版年画的发源地，朱仙镇木版年画诞生于唐代，兴盛于北宋，历经千年发展，至今依然广受欢迎。2006 年 5 月 20 日，朱仙镇木版年画经国务院批准列入第一批国家级非物质文化遗产名录。朱仙镇木版年画具有鲜明的地方特色，构图饱满，线条粗犷简练，造型古朴夸张，色彩新鲜艳丽，有别于历代文人画温文尔雅的艺术格调。朱仙镇木版年画艺术手法简洁明快，略带夸张，注重突出头部形象，身体比例夸张，

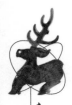

人物的面貌健美英俊而不带媚色。

朱仙镇年画源于民间，融入了民族传统文化的审美观念和原始崇拜，饱含人们爱憎分明的思想感情，也表达了人们希冀五谷丰登、富裕兴旺、平安吉祥的生活愿望。朱仙镇木版年画最常见的内容是门神，门神分文、武门神。文门神有五子、九莲灯、福禄寿等；武门神常是戏曲中的忠臣义士和各类英雄好汉，以秦琼、尉迟恭两位武将为主。此外，不同年龄的人房门上也会贴不同内容的门神：已婚子女的房门贴"天仙送子""连生贵子"，中年人房门贴"加官进禄""步步莲生"，老年人房门贴"松鹤延年"和寿星之类，少年人居室房门贴"五子夺魁""刘海戏金蟾"等。

Ⅲ. New Year Picture in Zhuxian Town

New Year picture, a kind of Chinese prints, originated from the ancient "Gate-God picture" and is one of the Chinese folk arts. It is often used in Spring Festival decoration, expecting good luck for the next year, building up an auspicious and festive atmosphere. Traditional folk New Year pictures are mostly made with technology of woodblock water-printing. The famous producers are Zhuxian Town in Kaifeng, Yangliuqing Town in Tianjin and Taohuawu in Suzhou.

As the birthplace of Chinese woodcut New Year pictures, Zhuxian Town's woodcut New Year prints were born in the Tang Dynasty and flourished in the Northern Song Dynasty. After thousands of years, they remain popular. On May 20th, 2006, Zhuxian woodcut New Year pictures were listed in list of the first batch of national intangible cultural heritage, approved by the State Council. Zhuxianzhen woodblock New Year pictures have distinctive features, full composition, rough and concise lines, simple and exaggerated modeling, fresh and gorgeous colors, which are different from the gentle artistic style of literati paintings in previous dynasties. The artistic techniques of Zhuxian Town woodcut New Year pictures are simple and vivid, highlighting the head and exaggerating the body proportion, with strong and handsome facial feature.

The New Year pictures of Zhuxian Town are originated from the folk, which have been integrated into the aesthetic idea and primitive worship of traditional national culture, and show people's love and hate, and express people's desire for a rich, peaceful life with good luck. The most common figures of Zhuxian Town woodcut New Year pictures are the Gate-Gods, which were divided into two groups, the god of civil servants and the one of military officer. The Gate-God of civil servant image often came from the stories such as *Five Sons with Promising Future*, *Lamp of Nine Lotus* and the images of the gods

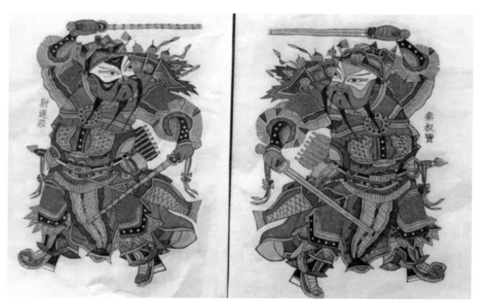

两位生活在 7 世纪的将军，左边是尉迟恭，右边是秦叔宝，通常作为所有人的保护者出现在新年木刻版画上。

These two generals lieved in the 7th century, Yuchi Gong on the left and Qin Qiong on the right, normally appearing on the New Year woodcut prints as everyone's protectors.

dominating good luck, fortune, and longevity. The gods of military officer are often loyal generals, righteous warriors or heroes, such as Qin Qiong and Yuchi Gong. In addition, the prints will vary from person to person of different ages. If someone gets married, they will choose the pictures related to babies, such as the pictures of "*Sending Children from the Heaven*". For the middle-aged people, they prefer prints suggesting good wishes of career. The door of old people's room usually is decorated with pictures about longevity and health. On the door of young people's living room, you will see pictures to wish them pass the most important exam.

参考文献

［1］刘玉梅.论中国传统木版年画的三大中心 [J].文化艺术研究，2021,14（04）:94−101.

［2］王树村.中国年画发展史.天津人民美术出版，2005.

实践活动

参观开封博物馆。

课后作业

在你的国家，人们怎么表达美好的祝福？

References

1.Liu, Yumei, *On the three centers of Chinese traditional woodblock prints for the New Year, Journal of Culture and artworks,* 2021,14(04)

2. Wang, Shucun, *The History of Chinese Traditional Prints for the New Year,* Tianjin Artworks Publishing House, 2005.

Activities

Visit the Kaifeng Museum

Homework

How do people extend wishes in your country?

四、开封汴绣

汴绣,起源于宋代都城开封,是当时手工业的一个重要行业。当时开封被称作"汴梁"或"汴京",这种刺绣也被称为"汴绣"。

汴绣以绣工精致、针法细密、图案严谨、格调高雅、色彩秀丽而著称,与苏绣、湘绣、粤绣、蜀绣一起合称为"中国五大名绣"。名绣各有所长,有的专精花鸟,有的长于虫鱼,而汴绣的题材多是仿绣古代书画作品,常见题材有书法、山水、花鸟、楼阁、人物等,其中尤以人物绣像最为突出。汴绣在表现形式上也深受中国画笔墨的影响,以绣线模仿绘画笔墨,用色厚重。汴绣有 36 种针法,技艺高超的绣工可以在一平方尺 0.11 平方米的绣布上绣 400 000 针,很多人都说这是指尖上的芭蕾。

清代以来,汴绣题材发生改变,以祝颂之辞和人物故事居多,如《群仙赐福》《百官上寿》《十八学士》等绣作皆有盛名。随后,汴绣绣品又出现了西洋风格的油画、装饰画、大型壁画等新型作品。

IV. Bianxiu in Kaifeng

Bianxiu, a kind of embroidery artworks with unique skill and style, originated from Kaifeng, the capital city of China in the Song Dynasty, was an important handicraft industry at that time. Kaifeng was called "Bianliang" or "Bianjing", so people name the embroidery works as "Bianxiu".

Bianxiu is famous for its exquisite workmanship, fine stitching, rigorous pattern, elegant style and beautiful colors. Together with Su (Suzhou, a city at southeast China) embroidery , Xiang(the abbreviation of Hunan Province) embroidery, Yue (the abbreviation of Guangdong Province) embroidery and Shu (the abbreviation of Sichuan Province) embroidery, they were known as "China's five famous embroidery artworks". Each of those five artworks has its own unique advantages. Some of them specialize in images of flowers and birds, while others are good at pictures of insects and fish. Bianxiu artworks choose to imitate calligraphy and painting works, including the Chinese Characters, mountains and rivers, flowers and birds, pavilions, figures, especially portrait paintings. Bianxiu was also greatly influenced by Chinese painting in terms of its expression. It imitates the ink color and shadow with various threads and superb crafts. Bianxiu has 36 stitching ways. The excellent artists can make around 400,000 stitches in each 0.1 square meter, so many people say this is the ballet on human's finger.

Since the Qing Dynasty, the theme of Bianxiu artworks have changed. Most of the artworks express best wishes or stories, such as "Blessings from Immortals", "Best Wishes from Officials", and "Eighteen Scholars". Later, in Bianxiu artworks also emerge western style oil paintings, decorative paintings,

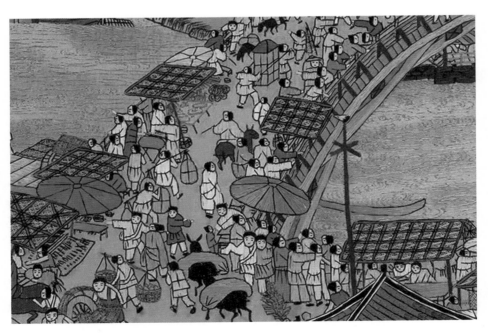

汴绣《清明上河图》（部分）

Bianxiu Artwork: "Riverside Scene of Qingming Festival" (part of the whole work)

large-scale murals and other new works.

五、灵宝剪纸

中国剪纸是一种用剪刀或刻刀在纸上剪刻花纹，用于装点生活或配合其他民俗活动的民间艺术。灵宝剪纸是指流传于河南省灵宝市的民间传统美术，其制作工艺简便，美观实用，深受广大群众喜爱。逢年过节，婚丧嫁娶，民间都要用剪纸布置居室，主要有窗花、棚花、炕屏、床围花、各种装饰花等等。

灵宝剪纸历史悠久。相传春秋时期，某年春节之后，灵宝桃林塞一带流行瘟疫，百姓苦不堪言。恰逢老子骑着一头神奇的青牛经过此地，老子非常同情当地人民，于是青牛口吐药物（中药牛黄），老子指导乡医将其分食于患者，疾疫随即散去，人们欣喜若狂，视青牛为救星。以后，每年正月二十三，家家都用黄棱纸剪金牛图贴在门上，意在避疫求吉，除恶压邪。此后，剪纸艺术流行于民间。

灵宝剪纸表现的内容丰富多样，花鸟草虫，人物走兽，千姿百态。灵宝剪纸善于使用谐音和寓意的手法来寄托人们对美好生活的向往。如：结婚布置新房就剪龙刻凤，寓意龙凤呈祥；剪莲花、石榴寓意连生贵子、多子多福等等；新春之际家家要贴双鱼、牡丹、大鸡等剪纸，寓意富贵、吉利、年年有余等。

V. Paper-cut in Lingbao County

Chinese paper-cut is a kind of folk art that uses scissors or knives to cut and carve patterns on paper to decorate life or cooperate with other folk activities. Lingbao paper-cut refers to the traditional folk art spreading in Lingbao County, Henan Province. It's simple to cut, which is beautiful, practical and popular among local people. For the Spring Festival, funerals, and wedding ceremonies, people use paper-cuts to decorate their rooms, mainly including showing on windows,

66

shed flowers, ornamental screen arranged on a heatable brick bed, bed surround flowers, all sorts of adornment flowers and so on.

Lingbao paper-cut has a long history. It is said that in the Spring and Autumn Period, the plague hit a small village, Taolinsai at Lingbao after the Spring Festival. People suffered a lot. It happened that Laozi, one of the most famous sages in Chinese history, passed by Taolinsai on a magic Ox's back. That magic ox spitted out a sort of medicine, calculus bovis, which cured the patients and stopped that epidemic. People were overjoyed and regarded that magic ox as the Savior. After that, every year on the 23rd day of the first month of Chinese Lunar New Year, local people used yellow edged paper to cut and paste pictures of Taurus on the door, in order to avoid the epidemic, pray for good fortune, eliminate misfortune and suppress evil. Since then, paper-cutting has been popular at Lingbao.

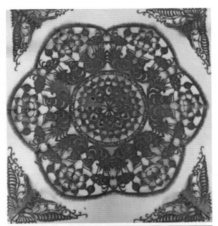

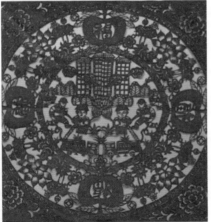

这些剪纸工艺品象征着人们对好运和幸福生活的期望。

The paper-cutting art crafts symbolize people's expectations for good luck and happy life.

Lingbao paper-cutting presents a variety of images, such as flowers, birds, grass, insects, characters, animals, and so on. It uses homophony and symbols to express people's yearning for a happy life. When people have the wedding ceremony, they will decorate the house with buy the images of Chinese dragon and phoenix, symbolizing that the couple will live a happy life. The image of lotus and pomegranate means to have many children. When the Spring Festival is coming, people will paste paper-cuts such as fishes, peonies and roosters, which mean to have wealth, auspiciousness and surplus year after year and so on.

实践活动

1. 参观灵宝。

2. 体验剪纸。

课后作业

介绍一下你们国家的手工艺术品。

Activities

1. Visit Lingbao County in Henan Province.

2. Experience paper cutting.

Homework

Share pictures about the famous handicrafts in your country with your classmates.

第六节　中原传统美食

一、河南烩面

河南面食多有所长。烩面是河南特色美食，它是一种荤、素、汤、菜、饭聚而有之的传统风味小吃，与北京的炸酱面、山西的刀削面、湖北的热干面、四川的担担面，同称为中国五大面食，享有盛誉。

郑州号称"烩面之城"，烩面馆遍布全市的华街冷巷。外地人来到郑州，首先想到的便是尝一尝地道的羊肉烩面，本地人款待亲朋的保留菜式也

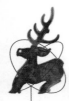
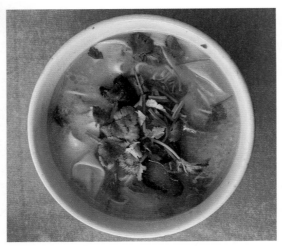

河南烩面
Henan stewed noodles

是香浓的烩面。

烩面是一种荤、素、汤、菜、饭兼而有之的河南传统美食，属于豫菜。河南烩面以优质高筋面粉为原料，辅以高汤及多种配菜，类似宽面条，以味道鲜美、汤好面筋、经济实惠、营养丰富享誉中原，遍及全国。烩面有羊肉烩面、三鲜烩面等多种类型，与胡辣汤、开封灌汤包并称为河南三大小吃。

河南烩面所用的面为扯面，一般用精白面粉，兑入适量盐碱和成软面，经反复揉搓，使其筋韧，揪成小剂子，捏成片状再两面摸上麻油。煮面之时，几番抖动，面片便由粗变细，被拉成宽约2厘米的薄面条，在滚水里浮沉几番也不易断开，面分为四两或二两一份。

烩面的精华全在于汤。羊肉汤要选用上好鲜羊肉，用反复浸泡后的上等嫩羊肉与羊骨（劈开，露出中间的骨髓）一起下锅，撇出血沫，放入全大料，加入党参、当归、黄芪、白芷、枸杞等七八味中药，既去了羊肉的膻气，又消减了羊肉的火气，十分滋补。先用大火猛滚，再用小火煲，煮五个小时以上，将肉煮烂，以把骨头油熬出来为佳，煲出来的汤白白亮亮，犹如牛乳一样，所以又有人称之为白汤。下面时，锅内放原汁肉汤，将面拉成薄条入锅，辅料有海带丝、千张丝、豆腐丝、粉条、黄花菜、木耳、香菜、鹌鹑蛋、海参、鱿鱼等，上桌时外带香菜、辣椒油、糖蒜、辣椒碎等小碟，其味更鲜。

Section VI Traditional Cuisine of the Central Plains

Ⅰ. Henan stewed noodles

Food made of flour in Henan has many recommendations. Stewed noodle is Henan's specialty, which is a traditional snack consisting of meat, vegetable, soup, and rice. It is also known as one of China's five major pastas and enjoys high reputation with fried sauce noodles in Beijing, sliced noodles in Shanxi, hot dry noodles in Hubei and Dandan noodles in Sichuan.

Zhengzhou is known as the "City of Stewed Noodles" with noodle restaurants occupying everywhere. When outsiders come to Zhengzhou, the first thing that comes to mind is to taste the authentic mutton stewed noodles. Locals would also cater relatives and friends with it as the reserved dishes.

Stewed noodles is a traditional Henan dish combing meat, vegetable, soup and vegetables, which belongs to Yu cuisine. It is made of high-quality and high-gluten flour with the appearance similar to fettuccine, and supplemented by stock and a variety of side dishes. It gains great reputation in the Central Plains and spreads throughout the country for its delicious taste, palatable soup, stretchy noodles, friendly price and rich nutrients. There are stewed noodles with mutton, seafood and many other types. It shares the title of "Three Famous Snacks of Henan" with spicy soup and Kaifeng soup dumplings.

Henan stewed noodles are generally hand-pulled with fine white flour. People add appropriate amount of saline to make the dough soft. Then they knead repeatedly to make it resilient. After divided into a few little doughs, each one would be pinched into flakes with both sides touched with sesame oil.

While cooking noodles, several shakes would make the noodles thinner with a width of about 2CM. The noodles are elastic enough to float and sink for a couple of times in the boiling water. Each portion of noodles is 100 or 200 grams.

The essence of stewed noodles lies in the soup. The mutton soup should be cooked with good fresh tender mutton and sheep bones (split to expose the middle bone marrow) that have been repeatedly soaked. Then, skim the blood foam from the soup and add seven or eight kinds of Chinese herbs, such as Dangshen (Chinese medicine), angelica, astragalus, the root of Dahurian angelica and medlars etc. Thus, it can not only remove the strong smell of the mutton but also cut down the internal heat inside and make the soup very nutritious. At the beginning, boil it with high heat. Afterwards, turn to low heat for more than five hours. It is better to boil the meat thoroughly so that it can leak the bone oil out. At last, the soup would be as white and bright as milk, which account for the name of "white soup". Next, pour the original broth in the pot and followed by the noodles pulled into thin strips. The auxiliary materials are shredded kelp, bean curd skins, shredded bean curd, vermicelli, daylily, agaric fungus, coriander, quail eggs, sea cucumber and squid, etc. To add some coriander, chilli oil, sugar garlics, chopped chili and other trimmings before serving would make it taste more delicious.

实践活动

1. 找寻郑州市烩面品牌店，了解烩面店文化。

2. 品尝河南烩面。

课后作业

小组讨论：品尝河南烩面后的感想。

Practical activities

1. Find the brand stores of stewed noodles in Zhengzhou and learn the culture of those stores.

2. Taste the Henan stewed noodles.

Homework

Group discussion: reflections of tasting Henan stewed noodles.

二、洛阳水席

说到洛阳的水席，可能没有来过河南的朋友会认为是一道菜，或者是一道小吃，其实不是的。洛阳水席是河南洛阳具有地方特色的传统宴席，属于豫菜系，是从唐朝开始流行的，到现在已经有着一千多年的历史了，是保留至今的名宴之一。在唐朝的时候，只有达官贵人才能吃到，比较贵，但是在现在基本上是经常可以吃到的，许多人朋友聚会、生日宴会等等宴请亲朋好友或者家里有喜事和大事都会吃到洛阳水席。

洛阳水席有两个含义：一是全部的热菜都有一些汤，含水量特别大，所以称为水席；二是吃完一道菜再上另一道菜，像流水一样不断更新，所以才称为水席。其特点是有肉有素，荤素搭配，材料比较多，由酸、甜、辣和咸组成。洛阳水席是24道菜组成的，分别是8道凉菜、16道热菜和汤。

8道凉菜又称为冷盘，分为四荤四素，做开胃菜和下酒凉菜，比较爽口和开胃。四盘素菜一般是凉拌莲菜、凉拌黄瓜、凉拌粉皮、凉拌芹菜、肉菜是五香牛肉、凉拌猪耳丝、鲟鱼和鸡柳。

16道热菜和汤也有荤有素，其中第一道菜是牡丹燕菜。关于牡丹燕菜还有个小故事，牡丹燕菜是用蛋黄做皮放在菜上，再加上红绿丝的搭配感觉就像黄帝的衣服一样。当时的女皇武则天在品尝过这道菜之后，感觉像吃了燕窝，还有它的寓意也是比较符合武则天气质的，所以赐名为燕菜。后来厨师在这道菜中用鸡蛋做了一朵牡丹花，所以被改名为牡丹燕菜，一直沿用到今天。

上了牡丹燕菜之后，接着上几道菜，鸡、鸭、鱼和肘子等肉菜为主，穿插着虾和几样汤，然后是八宝米饭和糖醋里脊等两道特色的甜汤。

不管席间的菜色怎么改变，起初的牡丹燕菜和最后的鸡蛋汤是不会改变的。其中的熬菜、连汤肉片、焦炸丸子汤、黄河大鲤鱼、小酥肉、海参汤等等都是比较出名的。

Ⅱ. Luoyang Water Banquet

As far as Luoyang water banquet is concerned, people who have never come to Henan may think it is a course or a snack, but it is actually a traditional banquet with local features in Luoyang City of Henan Province. It falls under the category of Henan cuisine and started to be popular in the Tang Dynasty, which is one of the famous banquets handed down till now, with a history of more than a thousand years. In the Tang Dynasty, Luoyang water banquet was only accessible to high officials and noble lords because of the high price, but now most people can have it frequently on the occasions of happy events or great events where lots of relatives and friends will be invited to celebrate such as gatherings and birthday parties.

Luoyang water banquet implies two meanings. First, there is soup in all hot dishes and they contain a great amount of water, so it is called "water banquet". Second, the dishes are served and updated one after another like running water, and this is the other reason why it is named "water banquet". Luoyang water banquet is characterized by a balanced mix of vegetables and meat and combined tastes of being sour, sweet, bitter andsalty, which is composed of twenty-four courses, including eight cold dishes and sixteen hot dishes and soup.

The eight cold dishes consist of four meat dishes and four vegetarian dishes that are served as appetizer and side dish for drinking because of the refreshing

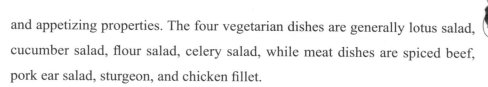

and appetizing properties. The four vegetarian dishes are generally lotus salad, cucumber salad, flour salad, celery salad, while meat dishes are spiced beef, pork ear salad, sturgeon, and chicken fillet.

The sixteen hot dishes and soup are also made of both meats and vegetables. The first dish served in a water banquet is "Peony Swallow Dish" and there is also a story about it. "Peony Swallow Dish" was made of an egg yolk sheet that was put on the vegetables and decorated with red and green strips, which looks like the clothes of the Emperor. At that time, Empress Wu Zetian felt that she had eaten the bird's nest after tasting the dish. Besides, its implied meaning was also in line with the temperament of Wu Zetian, and thus it was called "Swallow Dish". Later, the chef made a peony flower with eggs in this dish; therefore, it was renamed as "Peony Swallow Dish" and this name has been used till now.

After the "Peony Swallow Dish" is served, several other dishes and soup that are mainly made of chicken, duck, fish, pork joint and lobsters will be presented to you, followed by two special sweet dishes of eight-treasure glutinous rice and sweet and sour fillet of pork.

73

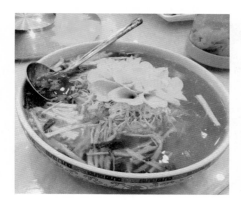

牡丹燕菜
Peony Swallow Dish

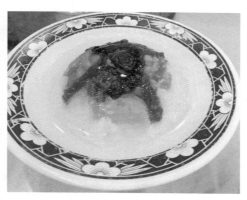

油炒八宝饭
Fried eight-treasure glutinous rice

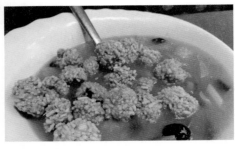

汆丸子

Quick-boiled meat balls with soup

No matter how the other dishes are changed, the first dish "Peony Swallow Dish" and the last course "egg soup" will never change. Among various dishes, "sliced meat with soup", "fried meatball soup", "Yellow River carp", "crispy meat" and "sea cucumber soup" are all very famous.

实践活动
到洛阳"真不同饭店"品尝洛阳水席，听服务员讲解每道菜品的典故，在品菜时了解洛阳兴盛。

课后作业
洛阳水席里你最喜欢的一道菜是什么？请配图并说明为什么。

Activity
Taste Luoyang water banquet, listen to the waiter/waitress to explain the allusion of each course, and get to know the prosperity of Luoyang while tasting the food in Luoyang "Zhenbutong" Restaurant

Homework
What is your favorite dish in Luoyang water banquet? Please illustrate the picture and explain the reason.

三、开封灌汤包

河南开封是一座文化古城，有着闻名世界的清明上河园，还有着享有"汴京富丽天下无"美誉的开封府。风景优美，历史悠久，开封整个城市都有着浓浓的历史韵味。除了深厚的文化底蕴，开封还有足够丰富

来华留学生中原中医药文化体验双语教程

A Chinese-English Course on Traditional Chinese Medicine for Foreign Students in China

的美食文化。除了鼓楼的夜市小吃，还有一种开封最出名的美食，它就是开封灌汤包。

开封灌汤包已有百年的历史，以纯正浓郁的汤和晶莹剔透的包子皮出名。正如它的名字一样，它的体型虽小，但是咬一口，它的汤汁立马涌了出来。甜咸正好的肉馅与汤汁和薄薄的馅皮在口中充分搅合在一起，令人心旷神怡，吸引了众多的食客。

蒸熟的汤包端上来，热气腾腾，雪白晶亮。拾箸夹起来，饱满得像盏小灯笼，隐约可见里面汤汁摇动，有一种吹弹就破的柔滑，不要说吃了，看着就是一种美的享受。对着一个个晶亮剔透的汤包，你可千万不要急着下口，否则热热浓浓的汤汁可要溅你一身。正确的方法：轻轻提起汤包上面的褶皱，细细地咬上一小口，拌着扑鼻香味，徐徐地吸吮粉红色的汤汁，顿觉唇齿留香，你再慢慢品尝汤包，浓香的肉馅配上筋道的包皮，令你食欲大增。

开封灌汤包不仅营养高，而且脂肪含量低，吃了健康不发胖！

Ⅲ. Kaifeng soup dumpling

Kaifeng in Henan Province is a city with ancient culture, where there is the world-renowned Millennium City Park and Kaifeng Prefecture that enjoys the reputation of "Bianjing being the most splendid city in the world". With a beautiful scenery and long history, Kaifeng is full of strong historical charm throughout the whole city. In addition to the profound cultural deposits, Kaifeng is also home to rich cuisine cultures, where there are not only night market snacks at the Drum Tower, but also the most famous delicacy—Kaifeng soup dumpling.

Kaifeng soup dumpling has a history of one hundred years, which is well-known for its pure full-bodied soup and crystal clear steamed stuffed bun skin. As the name suggests, although it is small in size, its soup will immediately gush out once it is bitten. The meat stuffing and soup with moderate sweetness and saltiness and the thinnish skin are fully mixed in the mouth, making people feel relaxed and happy; thus, it has attracted lots of diners.

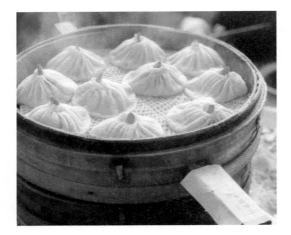

开封灌汤包

Kaifeng soup dumpling

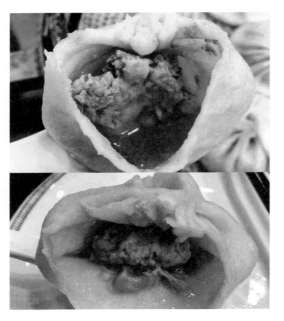

肉馅与汤汁

Meat stuffing and soup

Kaifeng soup dumplings are snow white and bright and steaming when they are served, which are very attractive. Each of them is very plump, just like a small lantern. When it is clipped up with chopsticks, you can faintly see the soup inside is shaking, and it is very soft and smooth as if it will break once it is blown by your mouth. Therefore, it is even a kind of enjoyment of beauty to just glimpse at it. In the face of the crystal-clear soup dumpling, you can never hurry to bite it; otherwise, the hot and full-bodied soup will splash you all over. The correct method is to slightly lift the wrinkle on top of the soup dumpling and then take a little bite carefully. Smelling the strong fragrance, you can insensibly suck the pink soup and enjoy the delicacy on your lips and teeth. Then, it is time to taste the dumpling with fragrant meat stuffing and chewy skin, which can greatly increase your appetite.

Kaifeng soup dumpling is not only high in nutrition, but also low in fat content. Therefore, it is a kind of healthy food which will not make you fat!

实践活动

到开封黄家老店品尝开封美食——灌汤包。若条件允许，可亲手试一试制作灌汤包。

课后作业

开封留给你印象最深的一道菜是什么？为什么？

Activity

Taste Kaifeng soup dumpling in Kaifeng Huangjia Laodian (a restaurant). If conditions permit, you can try to make the soup dumpling.

Homework

What is the dish that impresses you the most in Kaifeng? Why?

第七节　中原文化与发展成就实践

一、城市建设参观实践

得益于中原地区的强势崛起与快速发展，河南加大了城市建设力度，并且经过这些年的建设创新，更是取得了诸多令人称赞的优秀成果，比如郑东新区 CBD、洛阳洛邑古城等就是最具代表性的建筑，现已成为河南的新地标。

作为郑东新区的一个标志性建筑，CBD 利用两环 60 栋高层建筑组成环形城市，出于休闲、娱乐等考虑，还建设了具有一定规模的商业步行街及 24 小时不夜城。不仅如此，还在环形建筑群中间部署了河南艺术中心、会展宾馆等极具地标性的建筑物。

Section Ⅶ　Culture and Development Achievement Practice of the Central Plains

Ⅰ. Urban construction visit practice

Benefiting from the powerful rise and rapid development of the Central Plains, Henan has stepped up its efforts to conduct urban construction and achieved lots of complimentary excellent results through years of construction and innovation. For instance, the CBD in Zhengdong New District and Luoyang Luoyi ancient city are exactly the most representative buildings and have become the new landmarks of Henan Province.

As a landmark building in Zhengdong New District, CBD makes the advantage of 60 high-rise buildings in two rings to form a ring city. In consideration of the requirements for entertainment and leisure, a commercial pedestrian street with a certain scale and a 24-hour sleepless town have also been constructed. In addition, some other landmark buildings such as Henan Art Center and Exhibition Hotel have also been deployed in the circular building complex.

　　河南艺术中心建成以来，凭借浓郁的古典风格受到了人们的高度评价与深深喜爱。实际上这是国际知名大师卡洛斯・奥特根据河南出土的一些文物造型进行优化设计的，而艺术墙的灵感源于黄河翻卷的浪花造型。

Henan Art Center has been highly praised and deeply loved by people by virtue of its rich classical style since its completion. In fact, it was optimized and designed by the internationally renowned master Carlos Ott on the basis of the shapes of some cultural relics unearthed in Henan Province, while the inspiration of the art wall originates from the shape of the Yellow River spindrift when it is rolled up.

千玺广场的外形跟我们的农作物"玉米"非常相近，因此被人们形象地称为"大玉米"，它现在已凭借独特的圆形塔式设计风格成为标志性建筑。事实上，该建筑设计灵感源于古老的"嵩岳寺塔"，因此"大玉米"是历史的承载。

The appearance of Qianxi Square is very close to the shape of the farm crop "corn", and thus it is vividly called "big corn", which has already become a landmark building now by virtue of its unique circular tower design style. As

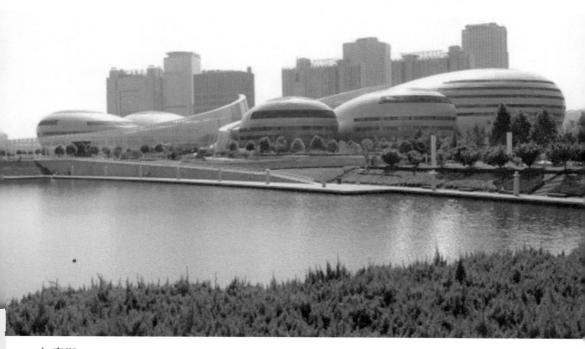

如意湖
Ruyi Lake

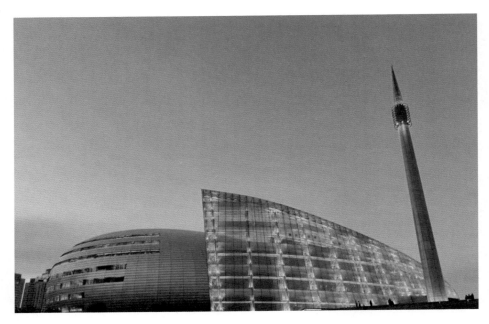

河南艺术中心
Henan Art Center

a matter of fact, this building was designed according to the inspiration arising from the ancient "Pagoda in Songyue Temple"; therefore, it can be said that "big corn" is a carrier of the history.

值得一提是，CBD 环形建筑群中间还专门设立了一个椭圆形的中心公园。中心湖能与湖泊公园连接，实现了船舶、游艇的自由穿梭。正是环形城市这一独特高层打造，使 CBD 成为最具国际特色的中心区。

What is worth mentioning is that an oval central park is specially designed in CBD circular building complex, where the central lake is connected to the lake park, thus realizing the free shuttle of ships and yachts. It is just because of the distinctive high-rise design of this ring city that makes CBD a central region with international characteristics.

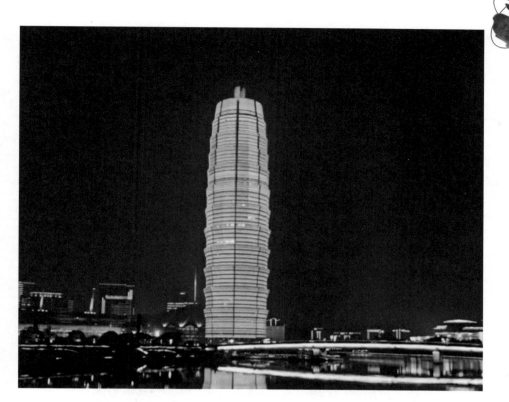

"大玉米"

"Big corn"

实践活动

参观郑东新区 CBD，感受郑州的日新月异。

课后作业

摄影展。请选出自己拍得最好的郑东新区 CBD 照片，大家比一比，看看谁的更好。

Activity

Visit CBD in Zhengdong New District and feel the rapid changes of Zhengzhou

Homework

Photography exhibition. Please choose the best CBD photos you take in

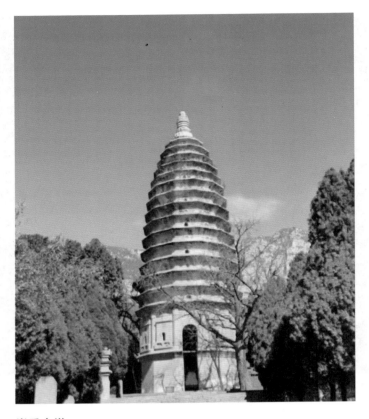

嵩岳寺塔
Songyue Pagoda

Zhengdong New District and compare which is better.

二、经济发展——大型工程参观实践

郑州奥体中心是极具特色的一个"地标性"建筑，无论是雄伟壮观的外观设计，还是功能化的内景部署，都可称为匠心之作，尤其是"一场两馆的"精心设计更是突出了它的独特性，而第11届全国少数民族传统体育运动会就是在此处举办的。

只要提到奥体中心，首先想到的就是"大"。据悉，郑州奥体中心融合了很多具有人文色彩且彰显地域特色的理念，而"天地之中、黄河天水"就是其中之一。体育场、体育馆、游泳馆的布局呈"品"形，不仅与黄河中的三座石岛相对应，而且附近环境也凸显了黄河水流动的盘旋性。奥体中心规模庞大、雄伟壮观，其占地面积超58万平方米。其中，体育场地上11层，凭借如此庞大的空间，实现了可容纳6万名观众同时观看的目的；体育馆地上4层，座席数量达到1.6万个；而游泳馆地上3层，其座席量设定为3 000个。它们具有规模大、配套全的优势，因此被定义为大型甲级场馆。

其次是功能全。"一场两馆"的独特设计可满足多种场景需求，比如综合性运动会、单项赛事等，地下还配套了集健身、娱乐、购物、住宿等多功能的大型商业区，可满足吃喝玩乐等多种需求。不仅如此，还专门打造了两层地下停车场，由此可最大化满足停车需求，根本不需要纠结停车问题，目前该停车场可同时满足3 950辆机动车、7 900辆非机动车停放需求。

对于容纳几万人的体育场馆来说，安全自然也是头等大事。实际上，早在设计初期，设计师就从安全角度进行了整体优化，而在建造过程中更是严抓结构、用料等事项，不用担心几万人聚集的安全问题。其中，"一场两馆"的钢材耗量高达4.7万吨，等同于一个"鸟巢"的规模。值得一提是，项目团队还将各种传感器部署在钢结构，通过在线监测系统的精准监测及时发现问题，由此保证了整套钢结构的性能优势。不仅如此，体育场馆内还设置了几百个疏散口，以加快人流疏散速度。比如仅在体育场三层看台就部署了66个疏散口，只需6 min就可实现所有人员的安全疏散。

‖. Economic development—large-scale project visit practice

Zhengzhou Olympic Sports Center is also an extremely characteristic landmark building. Either its magnificent appearance design or the functionalized interior deployment can be called a work of ingenuity, the meticulous design of "stadium+gymnasium and natatorium" especially highlights its uniqueness, and the 11th National Traditional Ethnic Minority Sports Games were exactly held here.

Whenever Zhengzhou Olympic Sports Center is mentioned, what we can first think of is "that it is big". It is learned that Zhengzhou Olympic Sports Center integrates lots of humanistic concepts that manifest regional features, and "the Yellow River in the middle of heaven and earth" is one of them . The layout of the stadium, gymnasium and natatorium is in the shape of " 品 *pin* (taste)", which not only corresponds to the three stone islands in the Yellow River, but also highlights the spiraling of the water flow of the Yellow River. Being enormous and magnificent, Zhengzhou Olympic Sports Center covers an area of more than 580,000 square meters. Therein, the stadium is composed of 11 floors above ground, which realizes the purpose of allowing 60,000 spectators to watch simultaneously by virtue of such a large space design. The gymnasium consists of 4 floors above ground with the number of seats up to 16,000, while the natatorium comprises 3 floors above ground where the number of seats is set at 3,000. Because of the advantages like great scale and complete supporting equipment, it is defined as a large-scale Class A venue.

The second feature is its complete functions. The specific design of "stadium+gymnasium and natatorium" can satisfy the needs of multiple scenarios, such as comprehensive sports meeting, individual sports event, etc. Besides, a large-scale multifunctional commercial zone that integrates fitness, recreation, shopping and accommodation is also equipped underground, satisfying people's needs in eating, drinking and entertainment. Furthermore, a two-story underground parking is specially created to meet people's parking demand to the maximum extent, so that you do not need to bother about the parking problem at all. At present, 3,950 motor vehicles and 7,900 non-motor vehicles can park in the lot simultaneously.

With regard to the stadium that accommodates tens of thousands of people, safety is naturally a matter of primary importance. In fact, designers performed overall optimization from the perspective of safety early in the design stage and paid much attention to the structure and materials in the process of construction. Therefore, there is no slight need for us to worry about the safety issue of tens of thousands of people gathering here. The steel consumed for building "stadium+gymnasium and natatorium" is as high as 47,000 tons, equivalent to the size of a "Bird's Nest". It is worth mentioning that the project team has also deployed various sensors in the steel structure so as to find the problem in time through the accurate monitoring of the online monitoring system and further ensure the performance advantage of the whole set of steel structure. What's more, the stadium is also equipped with hundreds of crowd exits to expedite the evacuation of people. For example, the spectators' stand on the third floor of the stadium is deployed with 66 exits and all people can be

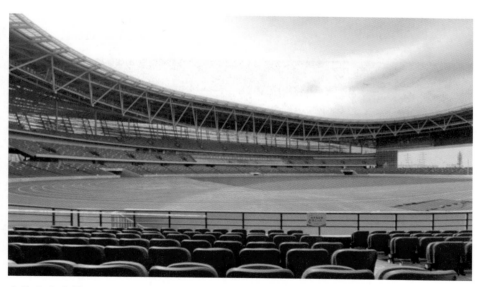

奥体中心内景
Interior of Zhengzhou Olympic Sports Center

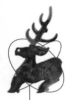

evacuated safely just within 6 minutes.

实践活动

参观郑州奥林匹克体育中心，了解建筑设计与中原地区的人文地理的密切关系。

课后作业

你知道南水北调工程吗？请上网查阅资料，南水北调工程涉及河南的什么城市？

Activity

Visit Zhengzhou Olympic Sports Center to learn the close relationship between architectural design and human geography in the Central Plains.

Homework

Do you know the South-to-North Water Diversion Project? Please look up information online to find out which city in Henan Province is involved in the South-to-North Water Diversion Project.

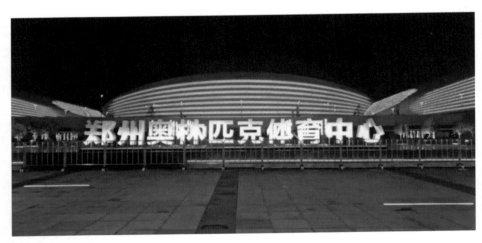

奥体中心夜景

Night scene of Zhengzhou Olympic Sports Center

第二章　中医药文化体验与实践

第一节　中原中医文化发源与历史

　　河南地处中原，位于中国中部的黄河中下游地区，在中国历史上长期占据政治、经济、文化的核心地位，是华夏文明的重要发祥地。在几千年的生产生活中，这里的世代居民不仅创造了文明奇迹，也创造了灿烂的中医药文化。在华夏文明进步与发展中，中医药不断地汲取营养逐步形成了独特的医药体系，中医药文化是传统文化中的精华部分，也是中国的国粹。在历史上，河南中医药对中华民族的繁衍昌盛做出了卓越贡献，对整个人类健康和世界文明产生了积极的影响，是中华医药文化的根基和主体。

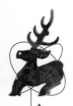

Chapter II   Experience and Practice of the Traditional Chinese Medicine

Section I   Origin and History of the Traditional Chinese Medicine in the Central Plains

Henan is located in the Central Plains, one of the main birthplaces of Chinese civilization. In thousands of years of production and life, people have not only created a miracle of civilization, but also created a brilliant culture of traditional Chinese medicine. In the development of Chinese civilization, Chinese medicine has formed a unique medical system, turning into the essence of traditional culture. Historically, Chinese medicine in Henan Province has made great contributions to the prosperity of the Chinese people, and has a positive impact on human health and world civilization. It is the foundation and main body of Chinese medicine culture.

一、中医药文化起源于中原

中国人常说"民以食为天""国以粮为本",农业在中国古代是非常重要的,也是世世代代中国人生存繁衍的前提。中原位于黄河中游地区,春夏秋冬四季分明,冷热适宜,河流众多,气候温和,土地肥沃,为农耕文化的发展提供了良好条件，从而也造就了中原人民的繁荣昌盛。在漫长的生活和劳动实践中，中原先民们逐步认识自然，从农耕生活经验总结出来指导中原人耕作和生活的二十四节气，还发现了能缓解病痛的动植物，逐渐用于治病及疗养，慢慢有了医药活动，后来又发明了针法、灸法和外治法等，留下了很多有关医药起源的传说，如伏羲"制九针"、神农"尝百草"等。夏商周时期，"伊尹创制汤液"改变了人们的用药习惯，开阔了用药领域，丰富了医药学知识和治疗方法，也为战国以后中医学理论的形成打下了基础。这些都充分说明河南是中医药的重要发祥地，中医药的源头在中原。

I. Chinese Medicine Culture Originated in the Central Plains

The ancient Chinese society was based on agriculture. The Central Plains meet the middle reaches of the Yellow River, with four distinct seasons, mild climate, vast plains, fertile soil and rivers system, which benefits a lot to agricultural culture. In the long time of life and working, early Chinese people understood the nature, finding animals and plants that could alleviate pain or have other medical impacts, which were considered as primitive medical activities. Later, they invented acupuncture, moxibustion and external treatment, leaving many legends about the origin of medicine, such as Fuxi's "Making Ninew Noodles" and Shennong's "Tasting Hundreds of Herbs". During the Xia, Shang and Zhou dynasties, Chinese medicine grew much faster. Yiyin, a famous chef and premier of the Shang Dynesty, cooked the herbal medicine as a sort of soup that is decoction we know today, which greatly changed people's medication habits, extended the medication activities, and broadened medical knowledge and treatment methods. This also laid a foundation for the formation of TCM theory after the Warring States Period. All of these have shown that Henan is an important birthplace of traditional

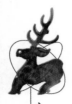

Chinese medicine. The source of traditional Chinese medicine is in the Central Plains.

二、中医药科学发达于中原

在中国的战国、秦、汉及三国时期（距今 2 500 到 1 800 年前），中国医学家，把阴阳五行学说中的朴素唯物主义思想和古代辩证法思想用于中医学的说理，把道家思想中的精、气、神等概念和摄生的论点引入中医学重要理论构建中；同时，中国儒家"仁义道德"思想中进步的内容，也对医学伦理学发展有积极作用。随着中医基础理论不断发展积累，《黄帝内经》《伤寒杂病论》和《神农本草经》等中医药学经典著作相继在中原地区完成并问世。《黄帝内经》奠定了中医理论的基础，成为后世中医理论之源；《伤寒杂病论》创立了辨证论治原则，完备了理法方药的理论体系，书中记载的方药被后世的中医大幅尊为经方，在唐代《伤寒杂病论》传入了日本、朝鲜、越南等国，在日本尤为医生推崇；《神农本草经》记录了药物学知识，提出了中药学"四气五味""君臣佐使"等理论。这些都对中医药理论的形成、丰富和发展起到了极其重要的作用。可以说中医药理论在中原形成，中医药经典在中原诞生。

唐代医家孙思邈，也曾长期在中原地区行医，著有《千金要方》《千金翼方》，集方剂之大成，使医学理论和医圣文化得以广泛传播。

宋金元时期，是中医药学发展的兴盛时期，医疗制度和设施逐步完善。北宋都城在开封设立"翰林医官院""太医局""御药院""尚药局""医药惠民局"等医政、保健、药政等机构。宋代医家王惟一，发明并铸造了针灸铜人，将针灸的临床与教学结合起来，为针灸学的发展和医学教育做出了巨大贡献。开封的"针灸铜人"是世界针灸医学发祥地的象征。

II. Chinese Medicine developed in the Central Plains

During the Warring States Period, the Qin Dynasty, the Han Dynasty and the Three Kingdoms Period, Chinese medical scholars combined the primitive materialism and dialectics into the theories of *yin-yang* and five elements, which were used as analyzing tools for the traditional Chinese medicine. Then people merged the concepts of essence, *qi* and spirit in Taoist thoughts and transplanted the argument of birth into the traditional Chinese medicine, while some of the ideas rooted in Confucian theory, like "benevolence, righteousness and morality", also play a positive role in the development of medical ethics. With the continuous development and accumulation of basic theories of traditional Chinese medicine, classic works of traditional Chinese medicine such as *Huangdi Neijing (Huangdi's Internal Classic)*, *Shanghan Zabing Lun (Treatise on Cold Damage and Miscellaneous Diseases)* and *Shennong Bencao Jing (Shennong's Classic of Materia Medica)* have been completed and published in the Central Plains. *Huangdi Neijing (Huangdi's Internal Classic)* laid the foundation of TCM theory and became the source of TCM theory in later generations. *Shanghan Zabing Lun (Treatise on Cold Damage and Miscellaneous Diseases)* established the principle of treatment based on syndrome differentiation and completed the theoretical system of principles, methods, formulas and medicinals. The prescriptions contained in it were respected as classical formula. In the Tang Dynasty, *Shanghan Zabing Lun (Treatise on Cold Damage and Miscellaneous Diseases)* was successively introduced into Japan, Korea, Vietnam and other countries, especially worshipped by doctors in Japan. *Shennong Bencao Jing (Shennong's Classic of Materia Medica)* records the herbal's knowledge, and puts forward the theories of four properties and five flavors of traditional Chinese medicine, and the ideas about the collocation of the formula. Zhang Congzheng founded the theory of purgation, as one of the four masters of the Jin and Yuan dynasties. All these have played an extremely important role in the process of developing

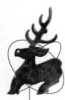

traditional Chinese medicine theory. It can be said that the theory of traditional Chinese medicine was born and formed in the Central Plains.

Sun Simiao, a physician in the Tang Dynasty, also practiced medicine in the Central Plains for a long time. His works, *Invaluable Prescriptions for Ready Reference* and *Supplement to Invaluable Prescriptions for Ready Reference,* collected the great achievements of prescriptions, so that the medical theory and medical sage culture could be widely spread.

During the Song, Jin and Yuan dynasties, TCM experienced a prosperous time .The medical administration facilities were gradually improved. The capital city of the Northern Song Dynasty set up medical administration, health care, pharmaceutical administration and other institutions in Kaifeng, such as "Hanlin Medical Officers' Bureau", "Imperial Medical Bureau", "Medical Administration Bureau", "People-benefiting Medical Bureau". Wang Weiyi, a physician in the Song Dynasty, invented and cast the bronze man of acupuncture and moxibustion, combined the clinical and teaching of acupuncture and moxibustion, and made great contributions to the development of acupuncture and moxibustion and medical education. The "bronze man of acupuncture and moxibustion" in Kaifeng is a symbol of the birthplace of acupuncture and moxibustion in the world.

三、中医药大师荟萃、名胜遍布于中原

中原历代名医辈出，人才荟萃，是对中医药学发展贡献最大的地区。据不完全统计，春秋战国至明末，史传中有籍可考的全国5 000多位名医中，河南就有912人。最著名的东汉时期南阳人张仲景，开办证论治之先河，被后世尊为"医圣"。宋金元时期河南民权人张从正是金元四大家之一，为中医"攻下派"的代表；河南许昌人滑寿在经络理论研究上的成就，对后世针灸学的发展产生了巨大的影响。明清时期，河南固

始人吴其浚编著了我国第一部大型植物志《植物名实图考》；河南孟津县的平乐郭氏正骨以其独特的理论和治疗技术，丰富了中医药文化宝库。此外，还有大批长期在中原地区从事医药活动的大家，如战国时期的神医扁鹊，三国时期外科鼻祖华佗，南北朝时期针灸家皇甫谧等，都曾在河南行医采药或著书立说。

南阳医圣祠、洛阳龙门药方洞、药王庙、十三帮会馆、神农涧等名胜古迹及开封"针灸铜人"都见证了中原医学文化的源远流长与博大精深。在仲景故乡河南南阳，人们为了纪念医圣，在清代建造了医圣祠。医圣祠作为供奉、纪念张仲景的场所，每年的祭祀活动都在这里举行，既有医药学家的朝圣祭祀，义诊施药，也有医林会馆的学术讲堂、座谈交流，还有当地百姓祭拜问药，祈福纳祥，亦有儒家文人的赋诗颂歌，已成为蔚为壮观的文化现象。国外的医家学者还专程到南阳拜谒医圣祠，将此称为"归宗"。可见中原医学文化的魅力和影响。洛阳龙门石窟的"药方洞"，保留有北齐时期完整的中医药方 118 个，治疗的病种达 37 个。这些药方为中国现存最早的石刻药方。

III. Masters and Monuments in the Central Plains

There have been a large number of famous doctors in the Central Plains. It is the area that has made the greatest contribution to the development of traditional Chinese medicine. According to incomplete statistics, from the Spring and Autumn period and the Warring States period to the late Ming Dynasty, there were 912 famous doctors in Henan Province. Zhang Zhongjing, the most famous person of Nanyang in the Eastern Han Dynasty, pioneered syndrome differentiation and treatment, and was respected as a "medical saint" by later generations. During the Song, Jin and Yuan dynasties, Zhang Congzheng, a civil rights man in Henan Province, was one of the four great masters in the Jin and Yuan dynasties and the representative of the "purgation school" of TCM. Hua Shou, who lived at Xuchang, a city in Henan Province, made great achievement in the study of meridian theory which had a great impact on the development of acupuncture and moxibustion. During the Ming and Qing dynasties, Wu Qijun, a native of Gushi County in Henan Province, compiled the first national flora of China, *Zhiwu Mingshi Tukao* (*Illustrated Reference of Botanical Nomenclature*). In Pingle of Mengjin County, Guo's bone setting enriched the TCM theory with its unique theory and treatment skills. In addition, there are a large number of people who have been engaged in medical activities in the Central Plains for a long time, such as Bian Que, a miraculous doctor in the Warring States period, Hua Tuo, the founder of surgery in the Three Kingdoms period, and Huangfu Mi, an acupuncturist in the northern and Southern dynasties. They all practiced medicine and gathered herbs and wrote books in Henan.

Nanyang Medical Saint Shrine, Luoyang Longmen Prescription Cave, the King of Medicine Temple, the Chamber of Thirteen Herbals Is Commerce Group, Shennong's Valley and other historical and cultural sites, as well as Kaifeng "bronze man of acupuncture and moxibustion" have all witnessed the long history and broad and profound medical culture of the Central Plains. In Nanyang, Henan Province, Zhongjing's hometown, people built a Medical Saint Temple in the Qing Dynasty to commemorate this great doctor. As a place to worship and commemorate Zhang Zhongjing, the medical shrine holds activities here annually, offering sacrifice and holding free clinic, academic activities, local people's praying for blessings and luckiness, as well as scholars' composing poems and Carols, which has become a phenomenon. Foreign doctors and scholars also make a trip to Nanyang to pay homage to the medical shrine, which is called "Guizong". It can be seen the charm and influence of the Central Plains medical culture. The "prescription cave" in Longmen Grottoes in Luoyang retains 118 complete traditional Chinese medicine prescriptions in the Northern Qi Dynasty, treating about 37 diseases, which are the earliest existing stone prescriptions in China.

四、道地药材盛产于中原

河南中草药资源十分丰富，盛产 2 780 多种中药材。产于焦作的"四大怀药"距今已有 3 000 多年的栽培历史。四大怀药是指在河南省焦作市所产的山药、牛膝、地黄、菊花等四大中药。自周代开始，历朝都将"四大怀药"列为皇封贡品。此外，河南还是禹白芷、裕丹参、密二花、息半夏、桐桔梗、山茱萸、辛荑花、连翘、冬凌草、柴胡等药材产地，药材道地，质优量大。

河南是中药材重要集散地之一。历史上有禹州、百泉两大全国性中药材交易会。春秋战国时期，禹州就有中药材交易活动和医家药商的会聚，明洪武年间形成规模，清乾隆年间药交会规模进一步扩大，全国各地药商多在此建立药行。百泉药会起源于隋朝，会期一个多月，日流量上万人。素有"春暖花开到百泉，不到百泉药不全"之美誉。

禹州的中药材加工、炮制始于明代，荟萃了历代技艺，因药制宜，技艺独特，制作精细，注重药效，在"浸、泡、锻、煨、炒、炙、蒸、煮"等方面形成了独特的地方特色。在 1911 年的"万国医药博览会上"禹州的"九蒸熟地"引起轰动。许多加工炮制技艺被载入经典。业内有"药不过禹不香"之说。

百泉药会、禹州的中医药材市场目前仍是中原中药材的非常有影响力的交流交易会。

IV. Genuine Regional Herbal Medicine are abundant in the Central Plains

Henan is rich in Chinese herbal medicine resources, abounding with more than 2,780 kinds of Chinese herbal medicines. "The Four Prestigious Herbal Medicines at Huaiqing", including Shanyao (Common Yam Rhizome; Dioscoreae Rhizome), Niuxi (Twotoothed Achyranthes Root; Achyranthis Bidentatae Radix), Dihuang (Rehmannia Root; Rehmanniae Radix) and Juhua (Chrysanthemum Flower; Chrysanthemi Flos) have been cultivated in Jiaozuo, a city at Henan Province for more than 3000 years. Since the Zhou Dynasty, "The Four Prestigious Herbal Medicines at Huaiqing" have been listed as imperial tribute in dynasties. In addition, Henan is also the excellent origin of many medicinal materials with good efficacy and high yield, including Yu Baizhi (Dahurian Angelica Root; Angelicae Dahuricae Radix) of Yu Zhou, Yu Danshen (Danshen Root; Salviae Miltiorrhizae Radix et Rhizoma) of Yu Zhou, Mi Erhua (Japanese Honeysuckle Flower; Lonicerae Japonicae Flos) of Xin Mi, Xi Banxia (Pinellia Tuber; Pinelliae Rhizoma) of Xi Xian, Tong Jiegeng (Platycodon Root; Platycodonis Radix) of Tongbai, Shanzhuyu (Asiatic Cornelian Cherry Fruit; Corni Fructus), Xinyi Hua (Biond Magnolia Flower; Magnoliae Flos), Lianqiao (Weeping Forsythia Capsule; Forsythiae Fructus), Donglingcao (Blushred Rabdosia Leaf; Rabdosiae Rubescentis Herba) and Chaihu (Chinese Thorowax Root; Bupleuri Radix), etc.

Henan is one of the important distribution centers of traditional Chinese medicine. The two national Herbal medicine fairs in history were located at Yuzhou and Baiquan. During the Spring and Autumn and the Warring States periods, Yuzhou gathered doctors and drug merchants to buy or sell Chinese herbal medicine. During the Hongwu years of the Ming Dynasty, the trading activities had wide impact widely. During the Qianlong's reign of the Qing Dynasty, herbal medicine merchants from all over the country established TCM pharmacy here. Baiquan's Medical Fair started from the Sui Dynasty, with a duration of more than one month and a daily flow of tens of thousands of people. People often said "When the spring is coming, people should go to Baiquan, otherwise one cannot collect all the herbal medicines he needs."

The processing of traditional Chinese medicine in Yuzhou began in the Ming Dynasty and gathered the skills of previous dynasties, undertaking the unique technology and fine production based on the different situations of herbal medicines, which product with good efficacy. It has formed unique local characteristics in the processing skills like "dipping, soaking, burning, baking, frying, roasting, steaming and boiling". In 1911, the skill of "steaming Shudihuang (Prepared Rehmannia Root; Rehmanniae Radix Praeparata) for nine times" from Yuzhou's herbal processor caused a sensation at the "World Medical Expo". Many processing techniques have been recorded in classics. There is a saying in this industry that "Medicine is fragrant only after it is processed at Yuzhou".

Pharmaceutical Fairs at Baiquan and traditional Chinese medicine market at Yuzhou are still very influential commercial activities of traditional Chinese medicine in the Central Plains.

五、中原中医药历史悠久

从原始社会到现代的历程中，中原中医药经历了酝酿、萌芽、诞生、成熟、繁荣和复兴的发展阶段，形成了底蕴深厚的河南中医药文化。

河南是历史文化大省，在50万年以前已经有了古代先民的生活足迹，大量的古人生活遗迹显示，人们已经会用火来烧制陶器，建筑房屋，发明使用最早的医疗用具——砭石（有锐利的尖端或锋面，手术刀、针的雏形），积累了丰富的卫生保健经验，为后来河南中医药的萌芽奠定了坚实的基础。

夏商周时期，文字开始出现。从《诗经》《山海经》等文献中，可以看到当时河南中医药的发展，人们对疾病的治疗、药物的使用已经积

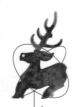

来华留学生中原中医药文化体验双语教程

A Chinese-English Course on Traditional Chinese Medicine for Foreign Students in China

98

累了一定的经验。这个时期中医的发展有两个重要的标志事件，分别是酒和汤剂的创制。

出土于河南新郑的"莲鹤方壶"是春秋时期的青铜礼器，用来盛酒。人们在长期饮酒中发现了酒的药用功效，它可以祛风散寒，活血通络，消除疲劳，所以酒被逐渐应用到中药领域当中，后世把酒的右半边"酉"字借鉴过来组成了"醫"的下半边。

出土于河南郑州的"杜岭方鼎"是商代早期的青铜鼎，是从陶鼎演变过来的。把煮饭用的鼎做得这样精美，说明当时中原人对饮食烹饪的工艺已掌握得十分精巧，也足以支撑证明商代是可以创造出"汤剂"这种东西的。伊尹在长期烹调的过程中发现，不仅食物在煎煮过程中味道会发生变化，同样，药物在煎煮的过程中既能被消毒杀菌，也会发生一些奇妙的变化。对于中医来讲，汤剂的发明具有跨时代意义。

中原哲学思想十分丰富，《周易》的阴阳思想和《尚书》的五行学说对于中医理论体系的构建起到了奠基作用，而老子、庄子的道家思想以及墨子、韩非子等人对中医养生学的形成也产生了很重要的影响。

南北朝隋唐五代时期，河南中医药名医辈出，留下了丰富的

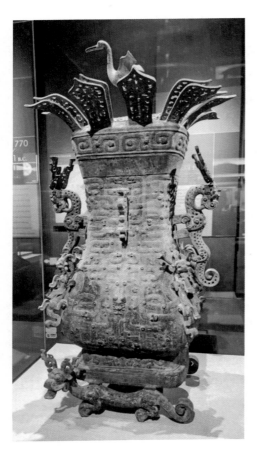

莲鹤方壶
The Square Lotus Crane Pot

医学著作，如《褚氏遗书》《食疗本草》《古今录验方》，尤其是《古今录验方》，里面关于"糖尿病病人的尿液是甜的"记载是世界上最早的。唐代诗人刘禹锡所著《传信方》一书所载方剂多为简便廉验之方，在国内外产生了重要影响，为医学事业也做出了很大的贡献。

宋金元时期，北宋末年南宋初年河南籍的宫廷画家李唐所绘制的"艾灸图"（又名村医图），是反映中医药为主的一幅名画，以村医为老翁治病为素材进行创作，表现了一个普通民间医疗的

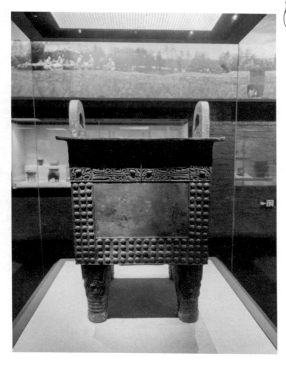

杜岭方鼎

Duling square tripod

99

场景：在一家小院中，一位民间医生正在给一个病人做艾灸和切除表面疮疡的手术，旁边还有一个助手准备帮病人贴膏药。

北宋的都城在河南开封，是全国的政治、经济和文化中心，也是医学中心，当时政府对医学十分重视，有利于中医的发展。当时的印刷术发展迅速，对于医学文献的整理、流传来讲起到了重要的推动作用。政府主持督造了针灸铜人用于教学和考核。铜人的胸腹部可拆卸，拆卸完以后，内部是铜雕刻的脏腑，有利于当时的学生学习解剖等；而铜人的表面遍布了很多穴位，这些穴位可以容纳水和汞，在学生考试前，在穴位里灌入水或水银，考试的时候在表面涂上黄蜡，让学生进行针刺，如果针刺准确，水或水银就会流出，如果针刺错误，针就会弯掉。这是一

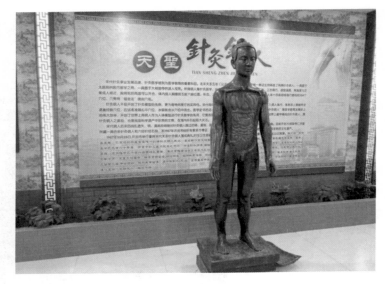

针灸铜人

Acupuncture bronze man

个很好的用于针灸考试和教学的用具。

　　宋朝名画《清明上河图》中有很多与中医药文化相关的遗迹，从图上能找到十余处药铺和诊所，甚至在一个十字路口就能找到三处中医药处所。其中最为明显的就是赵太丞家的专科诊所，它门前的招牌就是"治酒所伤真方集香药丸"，专门治疗喝酒所伤的肠胃病。北宋政府还设置医药惠民局，是采购药材、加工药材、销售药材的机构，保证了药材的纯正及质量，有利于临床医疗技术的提高。

　　明清时期，河南的中医药行业兴旺发达，诞生了很多名医和医学著作，像《救荒本草》《伤寒瘟疫条辨》等等都是具有代表性的著作。明清时期也为河南留下了三个国家级非物质文化遗产，分别是陈式太极拳、洛阳平乐郭氏正骨和四大怀药。

　　河南历史悠久，中医药文化底蕴深厚，有丰富的中医药文化遗迹，上至伏羲、神农、黄帝，下至张仲景、孙思邈，都是中医药文化的代表，如果有机会可以去相应的地方参观游玩。

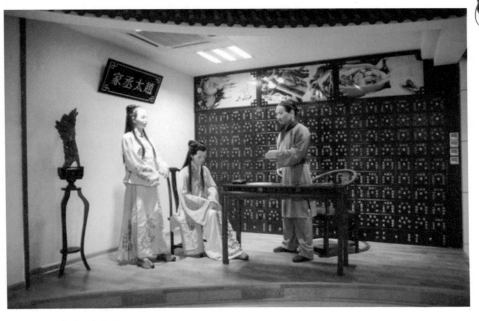

赵太丞家的专科诊所
Zhao Taicheng's specialist clinic

V. The Long History of TCM in Henan

From the primitive society to modern times, traditional Chinese medicine in the Central Plains has experienced the development stages of brewing, germination, birth, maturity, prosperity and rejuvenation, and formed a profound traditional Chinese medicine culture in Henan.

Henan is a province with long history and great culture. It has the life footprints of ancient ancestors 500,000 years ago. Among a large number of ancient life relics, people have been able to fire pottery, build houses, invent and use the earliest medical appliance—Bian stone (with a sharp tip or front, the prototype of scalpel and needle), and accumulated rich experience in health care. It laid a solid foundation for the germination of traditional Chinese

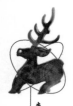

medicine in Henan.

During the Xia, Shang and Zhou dynasties, characters began to appear. According to *Shi Jing* (*Book of Songs*), *Shanhai Jing* (*Book of Mountains and Seas*) and other works, we can see the development of traditional Chinese medicine in Henan at that time. People have accumulated experience in diseases treatment and the use of drugs. In this period, the development of traditional Chinese medicine had two landmark events, namely, the creation of wine and decoction.

"Lotus Crane Rectangular Pot", unearthed in Xinzheng of Henan Province, is a bronze ritual vessel in the Spring and Autumn Period, which is used to hold wine. People have discovered the medicinal effect of wine which can dispel wind and cold, activate blood and dredge collaterals, eliminating fatigue. Therefore, wine has been gradually applied to traditional Chinese medicine. Later people take " 酉 ", part of the Chinese character of wine " 酒 *jiu* (wine)"as part of "medicine" 醫 .

The "Duling square tripod" unearthed in Zhengzhou, Henan Province is a bronze tripod in the early Shang Dynasty, which evolved from a ceramic tripod. The exquisite cooking tripod shows that people in the Central Plains had known a lot about cooking at that time, which proves that the Shang Dynasty could create "soup". In the long-term cooking process, Yi Yin found that boiling not only change the taste of food, but also disinfect drugs and stimulate some wonderful changes. For traditional Chinese medicine, the invention of decoction has cross era significance.

The Central Plains has many philosophy schools. The yin-yang thought in *Zhou Yi* (*Book of Changes*) and the five elements theory in *Shang Shu* (*Book of History*) have laid the foundation for the construction of the theoretical system of traditional Chinese medicine. The Taoist thought of Laozi and Zhuangzi and thoughts of Mozi and Han Feizi also had a very important impact on the formation of traditional Chinese medicine health preservation.

During the Southern and Northern Dynasties, Sui, Tang and Five Dynasties, Henan's famous TCM doctors came forth in large numbers, leaving behind a wealth of medical works, such as *Chushi Yishu* (*Fragmentary Book of Master Chu*), *Shiliao Bencao* (*Materia Medica for Dietotherapy*), *Gujin Lu Yanfang* (*Records of Effective Formulas of the Ancient and Modern Times*). The earliest record of the sweet urine of diabetics was in *Gujin Lu Yanfang* . Most of the simple and inexpensive formulas were contained in the book *Chuanxin Fang* (*Records of Effective Formulas*), written by Liu Yuxi, a poet of the Tang Dynasty. This book has made important impacts at home and abroad and made great contributions to medical science.

During the Song, Jin and Yuan dynasties, the Moxibustion Painting (also known as the Village Doctor Painting) drawn by Li Tang, a court painter from Henan in the late northern Song Dynasty and the early southern Song Dynasty, was a famous painting on Chinese medicine. It showed a scene of ordinary folk medicine: In a small hospital, a folk doctor is performing moxibustion and removing surface sores for a patient. Next to him, an assistant is going to paste a plaster for the patient.

Kaifeng of Henan Province was the capital of the northern Song Dynasty, which served as the political, economic and cultural center of the country, as well as the medical center. At that time, the government attached great importance to medicine, which was conducive to the development of traditional Chinese medicine. Printing technology developed rapidly at that time, which played an important role in promoting the collation and spread of medical literature. The government presided over and supervised the manufacture of acupuncture bronze men for teaching and examination. The chest and abdomen

103

of the bronze man could be disassembled, there was copper viscera inside. So it could help the students to know anatomy at that time. The surface of the bronze man was covered with acupoints. People could preserve water and mercury under the right point when the students took examination. During the examination, yellow wax was coated on the surface. If students could find right points, the water or Mercury would flow out. If the acupuncture was wrong, the needle would bend. So this was an excellent device for acupuncture examination and teaching.

Many relics related to TCM could be found in "The Riverside Scene at Qingming Festival", the famous painting of the Song Dynasty. More than ten medicine shops and clinics can be found on this painting, and even at one crossroad, three clinics can be found. The most obvious one is the specialist clinic of Zhao Taicheng's family. The shop sign went likes, Jixiang pill, a true useful formula for treating diseases caused by drinking alcohol, which specializes in treating gastrointestinal diseases caused by drinking. The government of the northern Song Dynasty also set up the People-benefiting Medical Bureau, which was an organization for purchasing, processing and selling medicinal materials, which ensured the purity and quality of medicinal materials and was conducive to the improvement of clinical medical technology.

During the Ming and Qing dynasties, the traditional Chinese medicine industry in Henan flourished, and many famous doctors and medical works were born, such as *Jiuhuang Bencao* (*Materia Medica for Famine Relief*) and *Shanghan Wenyi Tiaobian* (*Differentiation of the Cold Damage and Pestilence*). Since the Ming and Qing dynasties, three national intangible cultural heritages for Henan have been left, namely Chen Style Taijiquan, Guo's bone setting in Pingle of Luoyang and four prestigious herbal medicines at Huaiqing.

Henan boasts a long history of civilization, with great cultural heritages of traditional Chinese medicine. There are rich cultural relics related to TCM. From Fuxi, Shennong and Huangdi to Zhang Zhongjing and Sun Simiao, all of them are representatives of traditional Chinese medicine culture. If you have the chance, you can visit those places we have mentioned.

六、中医药博物馆参观与体验

河南中医药博物物馆位于河南中医药大学校园内，主要由河南医史馆、仲景馆、中药标本馆、中草药植物园等组成，是展示中原中医药历史及文化传承的窗口。

医史馆是河南省首家全面展示河南中医药发展历史的博物馆。建筑面积400余平方米，包括序厅、河南历代医史展和河南中医药文化遗迹展等3个主要展示区，共有古籍、青铜器、陶瓷、书画等各类藏品200余件。作为河南中医药博物馆的重要组成部分，医史馆有其丰富而厚重的展示内容、传统与现代相结合的展出形式，以及融中医药启蒙教育和中医药文化宣传于一体的功能，是社会大众了解中医、认识河南的重要窗口。

仲景馆是介绍张仲景生平及学术成就的纪念馆，有仲景的塑像，仲景塑像背后是小篆书写的《伤寒杂病论》，详细介绍了张仲景的生平、他的医学巨著《伤寒杂病论》以及仲景学术及流派的研究成就，仲景是中国医学史上的一座丰碑，是世界文明史上的人文地标！《伤寒杂病论》乃中医药学之基石，医学圣殿之瑰宝。仲景馆展示了中医药仲景文化的源远流长和博大精深。

中药馆面积600多平方米，主要展示了河南省生产的一些药用植物和中药材，反映了河南中药资源的基本概况。主要分为浸制标本展区、腊叶及生药标本展区和动物矿物药标本展区，各类标本2 800余份。其中的中药浸制标本，能完好地保持药用植物的茎、叶、花、果的原形、原色，使植物各部器官特征显而易见，把生长在不同地域、不同季节的药用植物集于一室，融知识性、教育性、科学性、艺术性于一体。植物腊叶标本是把采集带花或果的植物，在标本夹中压平、干燥后，装贴在台纸上，制作而成，供植物分类学研究使用。

"河南中药植物园"始建于 2014 年，占地面积 9.2 万平方米，共种植药用植物 500 余种，是集教学、科研、学生实践、种子种苗繁育、濒危中药资源保存、中医药知识普及于一体的多功能植物园。植物园一共划分为河南道地药用植物区、周边省份道地药材区、藤本药用植物区、水生药用植物区、观赏药用植物区、科研实验区、温室大棚育苗区、阴生药用植物区等八个区。

实践与学习任务

1. 参观河南中医药发展历史的博物馆。

2. 了解中医药文化元素的图片或雕像，如嵩山、黄河、河图洛书、伏羲画卦、甲骨文、八卦、神农、黄帝、伤寒论、张仲景以及针灸铜人等。

Ⅵ. Visiting the Museum of Chinese Medicine

Henan Traditional Chinese Medicine Museum is located on the campus of Henan University of Traditional Chinese Medicine. It is mainly composed of Henan Medical History Museum, Zhongjing Museum, Traditional Chinese Medicine Specimen Museum, Traditional Chinese Medicine Botanical Garden and other museums. It is also a window to show the history and cultural inheritance of traditional Chinese medicine in the Central Plains.

The Medical History Museum is the first one in Henan Province to display the history of traditional Chinese medicine. The floorage is more than 400 square meters, including three main exhibition areas: the preface hall, Henan Medical History Exhibition and Henan Traditional Chinese Medicine Cultural

Relics Exhibition. There are more than 200 collections of ancient books, bronze wares, ceramics, calligraphy and painting artworks. As an important part of Henan Museum of Traditional Chinese Medicine, the medical history museum will become an important window for the public to understand traditional Chinese medicine and Henan with its items on display, the combination of traditional and modern exhibition form, and the function of integrating Chinese medicine enlightenment education and traditional Chinese medicine culture publicity.

Zhongjing Museum is a memorial hall to introduce Zhang Zhongjing's life and academic achievements, with a statue of Zhongjing. Behind the statue is *Shanghan Zabing Lun* (*Treatise on Cold Damage and Miscellaneous Diseases*) written by small seal script Xiaozhuan, a special writing style of Chinese character, introduced Zhang Zhongjing's life, his medical masterpiece *Shanghan Zabing Lun* (*Treatise on Cold Damage and Miscellaneous Diseases*) and Zhongjing's academic achievements in detail. Zhongjing is a monument in the history of Chinese medicine, a cultural landmark in the history of world civilization. *Shanghan Zabing Lun* is the cornerstone of traditional Chinese medicine and the treasure of the temple of medicine. Zhongjing Museum shows the long history, the broad, profound Zhongjing culture of traditional Chinese medicine.

Covering an area of more than 600 square meters, the Traditional Chinese Medicine Museum mainly displays some medicinal plants and traditional Chinese medicine produced in Henan Province, reflecting the basic situation of traditional Chinese medicine resources in Henan Province. It is divided into immersion specimen exhibition area, wax leaf and crude drug specimen exhibition area and animal mineral drug specimen exhibition area, with more than 2,800 specimens. The soaked specimens can maintain the original shape and color of the stems, leaves, flowers and fruits of medicinal plants, so that the characteristics of each organ of the plant are obvious. The museum gathers the medicinal plants growing in different regions and seasons in one room, integrating knowledge, education, science and art. Plant wax leaf specimens are made by flattening and drying the collected plants with flowers or fruits in the specimen folder and pasting them on table paper for plant taxonomic research.

Henan Traditional Chinese Medicine Botanical Garden Chinese medicine botanical garden was founded in 2014, covering an area of 138 *mu* (a unit of area, which is equal to 0.0667 hectares) and planting more than 500 kinds of medicinal plants. It is a multi-functional botanical garden integrating teaching, scientific research, student practice, seed and seedling breeding, endangered traditional Chinese medicine resource conservation and popularization of traditional Chinese medicine knowledge. The botanical garden is divided into eight areas: Henan genuine medicinal plant area, periphery provinces genuine medicinal plant area, vine medicinal plant area, aquatic medicinal plant area, ornamental medicinal plant area, scientific research and experiment area, greenhouse seedling area and shade medicinal plant area.

Homework

1. Visit the Museum of History of Traditional Chinese Medicine in Henan.

2. Read the scenic spots, artworks or antiques related to traditional Chinese medicine, such as Songshan, the Yellow River, *Hetu Luoshu* (mystical diagrams symbolic of the universe and believed in myth to be related to the origins of writing), Fuxi painted hexagrams, oracle bone inscriptions, eight trigrams, Shennong, Huangdi, typhoid theory, Zhang Zhongjing, acupuncture bronze man, etc.

第二节　中医四诊

四诊是指望、闻、问、切四种中医诊察疾病的基本方法。

中医四诊即是通过望、闻、问、切四种方法来全面收集病人的症状和体征，以研究五脏六腑生理功能与病理变化在体表的表现，为疾病的诊断提供依据。

Section II　The Four Diagnostic Methods of Chinese Medicine

The four diagnosis methods are the four basic methods of Chinese medicine to diagnose and detect diseases by inspection, listening and smelling, interrogation, and palpation.

The four diagnostic methods of Chinese medicine is to comprehensively collect the symptoms and signs of patients through the four methods of inspection, smelling, inquiring, and cutting, in order to study the physiological functions and pathological changes of the internal organs on the body surface, and provide a basis for the diagnosis of the disease.

一、望诊

望诊是医生用视觉，对人体全部、局部及其自身的分泌物、排泄物等进行观察，以推断体内的变化。望诊在四诊中占有重要的地位，它可以帮助医者了解人体的精气盛衰、病情轻重、预后吉凶等，有"望而知之谓之神"的说法。因此，在就诊过程中，中医师首先通过望诊来判断疾病。主要包括望面色、望舌。

正常人的面色表现为红黄隐隐，明润含蓄，表示精神气血津液充盈，脏腑功能正常。若面呈白色，多为虚证、寒证；面呈红色，多为热证；面呈黄色，多属脾虚。

望舌主要察看舌质以及舌的形态、色泽、润燥等方面的变化。舌色淡红明润，柔软灵活，胖瘦老嫩适中，苔薄白，干湿适中，不黏不腻，为正常舌象。舌色淡白多为血虚、气虚、阳虚和寒证，舌红多为热证。

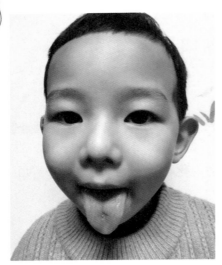

正常舌苔

The normal tongue

I. Inspection

Inspection refers to the observation of the whole and part of the human body and its own secretions and excretions by doctors with vision, so as to infer the changes in the body. Inspection plays an important role in the four diagnoses. It can help doctors understand the rise and fall of human essence and *qi*, the severity of the disease, and the prognosis. Therefore, in the process of treatment, traditional Chinese medicine doctors first judge the disease through inspection. It mainly includes inspection of complexion and tongue.

A ruddy complexion means that the spirit, *qi*, blood and body fluid are full, and the viscera function is normal. If the face is white, it is mostly deficiency syndrome and cold syndrome; if it is a red face, mostly it refers to heat syndrome; if it is a yellow face, mostly it belongs... to spleen deficiency.

Tongue inspection mainly observes the changes of tongue quality, shape, color, moistening and dryness. The normal tongue is light red, soft and flexible, with thin white coating. If the tongue… color is light and white, mostly there is blood deficiency, *qi* deficiency, Yang deficiency and cold syndrome; red tongue mostly represents heat syndrome.

二、闻诊

闻诊是医生用听觉和嗅觉诊察病人有关的声音和气味。

听声音指仔细听辨病人发声、语言、呼吸、咳嗽、呕吐等各种声响。若发声低微细弱，声音断续，多属虚证；呼吸气粗而快，属实证、热证；呼吸气微而慢，属虚证、寒证；干咳多见于津液不足，咳声低微属肺虚。

嗅气味指诊察病人散发出的气味以及分泌物、排泄物的气味。

如：口臭多见于胃气不和，如胃热、食积等；大便秽臭为热，酸臭多为伤食；小便黄赤浊臭，多属湿热。

II. Listening & Smelling

Listening and smelling is to detect the sound and odours of the patient.

Listening to sounds refers to carefully dividing the patient's voice, language, breathing, coughing, and vomiting. If the vocalization is low and weak, and the voice is intermittent, it is mostly a deficiency syndrome; thick and fast breathing is a positive heat syndrome; a slight and slow breathing is a deficiency or cold syndrome; a dry cough is more common in lack of body fluid, and a low cough is a lung deficiency.

Odor refers to the odor emitted by the patient and the odor of secretions and excreta. For example, bad breath is more common in stomach disharmony, such as stomach heat, food accumulation and so on. The foul smell of stool means a hot condition, while the sour smell means mostly food stagnation. If the urine is yellow, red, turbid and smelly, perhaps the person is in damp-heat condition.

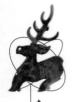

三、问诊

问诊是医生询问病人或陪诊者，了解疾病的发生、发展、治疗经过、现在症状和其他与疾病有关的情况，以诊疾病的方法。

主要包括姓名、年龄、性别、婚否、民族、职业、住址、家族史、既往史、起病、现在症状等。不同年龄、性别、职业、居住环境和就诊日期常常能提示好发病、多发病，比如工作环境潮湿，易中湿邪，还有职业病、地方病等。

Ⅲ. Interrogation

Interrogation is a way for doctors to ask patients or attendants to understand the occurrence, development, treatment process, present symptoms and other conditions related to diseases, so as to diagnose diseases.

Interrogation mainly includes asking the patient's name, age, gender, marriage, nationality, occupation, address, family history, past history, onset, present symptoms, etc. Different ages, genders, occupations, living environment and medical treatment dates can often prompt frequent diseases, such as humid working environment, easy to be infected with dampness. There are also occupational diseases and endemic diseases. Different ages, genders, occupations, living environment and medical treatment dates can often indicate frequently-occurring diseases, such as humid working environment, prone to dampness, and some occupational diseases and endemic diseases, etc.

四、切诊

切诊是用双手对病人肌体进行触、摸、按压，以诊察疾病的方法，主要包括脉诊和按诊两个部分。

Ⅳ. Palpation

Palpation is to touch and press the patient's body with both hands to diagnose the disease, mainly including pulse diagnosis and press diagnosis.

1. 脉诊

脉诊是四诊中发展较早的诊法，早在两千多年前，就已形成了比较完备的学说。临床常用的脉诊方法为寸口诊法。寸口脉位于前臂掌后拇指侧的桡动脉搏动处。定位方法：以桡骨茎突准确向内为"关"，关前（腕端）为"寸"，关后（肘端）为"尺"。两手各有寸、关、尺三部，计六部脉。左右寸口脉各有脏腑的归属：左寸候心与小肠，左关候肝与胆，左尺候肾与膀胱；右寸候肺与大肠，右关候脾胃，右尺候肾与命门。

1.Pulse diagnosis

Pulse diagnosis is one of the four early diagnostic methods. As early as 2000 years ago, pulse diagnosis has formed a relatively complete theory. Cunkou pulse diagnosis is commonly used in clinic: Cunkou pulse is located at the pulse of radial artery on the side of the thumb behind the palm of forearm. Positioning method: *Guan* is the inner position of the styloid process of radius; *cun* is before *guan* (wrist end); *chi* is after *guan* (elbow end). Each hand has three parts of *cun*, *guan* and chi, and six parts of pulse. Left and right *cunkou* veins have their own viscera: left cunkou for heart and small intestine, left cunkou for liver and gallbladder, left ulna for kidney and bladder, right cunkou for lung and large intestine, right cunkou for spleen and stomach, right ulna for kidney and mingmen.

2. 按诊

按诊手法包括触、摸、按等。其中，按肌肤以探明肌表的寒热、润燥以及肿胀；按手足以探明肌体的寒热；按腹以辨寒热、痛胀、肿块等；按腧穴可了解某些特定穴位是否有结节、条索状物、敏感反应，如压痛等，以了解相应脏腑及经络循行部位的病变。

2.Palpation

Palpation includes light touching, deep touching, pressing, etc. Palpating the skin can detect cold and heat, moisturizing and swelling of the body surface. Palpating hands is sufficient to detect cold and heat of the body. Palpate the abdomen can distinguish cold, heat, pain, swelling, etc. Palpate acupoints can understand whether there are nodules, cords, sensitive reactions, such as tenderness at certain specific acupoints, so as to understand the pathological changes of the corresponding viscera and meridian.

实践活动

1. 至中医养生馆脉诊参观体验。

2. 使用脉诊仪、面诊仪、舌诊仪实训体验，初步了解中医诊断原理。

Practical activities

1. Visit TCM Health Center and experience once pulse diagnosis.

2. Experience the pulse diagnosis instrument, face diagnosis instrument, and tongue diagnosis instrument, getting a preliminary understanding of the principles of TCM diagnosis.

第三节　中医药特色技术的体验与实践

一、针灸

针灸疗法是传统中医不可分割的一部分，有着悠久的历史。该疗法通过针或灸兴奋特定穴位以使失衡的机体恢复平衡态而治病防病。针灸起源于新石器时代，是世界最古老的医疗技术之一。16世纪针灸疗法从中国传入西方，于2010年11月16日被联合国教科文组织列入"人类非

114

物质文化遗产代表作名录"。

传统中医认为人体分布着复杂的网路，又称为经络，是能量（气）运行的通路，其阻塞将会导致机体失衡，进而引起各种疾病发生。针灸通过刺激体表的穴位，从而疏通经络，平衡机体，增强免疫力，以达到防病治病的目的。虽然针灸常常并称，但严格说来包括针刺与艾灸两部分。针刺利用各种头发粗细的针具刺入体表并辅以一定刺激如针刺手法或者仪器辅助，而艾灸则是燃烧艾绒或其他药物以达到刺激穴位治疗疾病的目的。

Section III　Experience and Practice of Characteristic Skills of Traditional Chinese Medicine

I. Acupuncture and Moxibustion

Acupuncture and moxibustion is an integral part of Traditional Chinese Medicine and has a long history. It uses acupuncture or moxibustion to excite specific points to restore the balance of the body and to cure and prevent diseases. This therapy originated in the Neolithic Age and is one of the oldest medical techniques in the world. It was introduced into the West from China in the 16th century and was listed in the "Representative List of the Intangible Cultural Heritage of Humanity" by the United Nations Educational, Scientific and Cultural Organization (UNESCO) on November 16, 2010.

Traditional Chinese Medicine believes that the human body is distributed with complex networks, which are also called meridians and are pathways of energy (*qi*) flow. The blockage of qi will lead to the imbalance of the body, and then cause various diseases. Acupuncture and moxibustion can dredge the

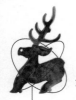

meridians, balance the body and enhance immunity by stimulating specific points on the body surface, which are also called acupoints, thus preventing and treating diseases. Although acupuncture and moxibustion are often referred to together, strictly speaking, it includes two different parts: acupuncture therapy and moxibustion therapy. Acupuncture therapy uses various hair-thin needles to penetrate the skin and assists the effect with certain stimulation, like manual manipulation or instrument stimulation; while moxibustion therapy burns mugwort or other herbs to achieve the purpose of acupoints stimulation.

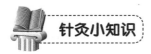 针灸小知识

针：最早的器具为砭石，即一端尖利的石块，可以刺激皮表穴位，同时也可用于外科化脓性感染的切开排脓。之后发展出"九针"，用于不同疾病的治疗。现代针刺疗法使用毫针居多，其规格不同，粗细长短各异，适于不同需求。例如无痛针细而软，面部美容多用；短针可用于耳针和手针；而长针则用于肌肉丰厚处。现代诸多研究表明，针刺可以通过影响神经、内分泌、免疫等系统治疗包括疼痛、压力、成瘾、肥胖在内的上百种疾病。

灸：字体可分解为"久""火"，其意为如火般长久温煦，具有温通经脉的作用。与自然界水流相似，能量网路（经络）在寒冷状态下流动凝滞，日久成疾。传统艾灸通过燃烧艾绒释放能量，刺激穴位，促进能量（气）在经络中流动，以恢复机体正常平衡状态。传统艾灸燃烧时会产生一定气味，一般认为这种气味对人体并无害处。现代也出现各种无烟艾，其具体疗效仍有争议。现代研究发现，艾灸可能是通过释放红外线的方式影响机体的。

Some knowledge about acupuncture and moxibustion:

Acupuncture: The earliest instrument was Bian stone, which has a sharp

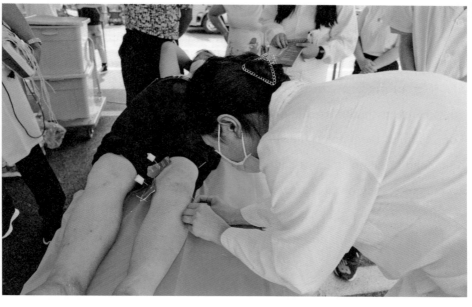

义诊现（艾灸）

Volunteer medical treatment—Moxibustion

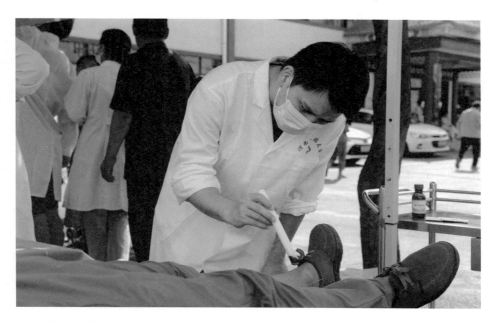

义诊现场（针刺）

Volunteer Medical Treatment—Acupuncture

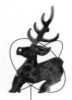
end, and can stimulate acupoints on the skin surface. At the same time, it can also be used for surgical incision and drainage in suppurative infection cases. Later on, the classic "Nine Needles" were developed for the treatment of different diseases. In modern times, filiform needles are mostly used, with different thicknesses and lengths, and are suitable for different needs. For example, the painless needle is thin and soft, and can be used for facial rejuvenation; short needles can be used for auricular acupuncture and hand acupuncture; long needles are used for areas with thick muscles. Many modern studies have shown that acupuncture can treat hundreds of diseases including pain, stress, addiction, obesity and so on by affecting the nervous, endocrine, and immune systems.

Moxibustion: The character "灸" can be divided into "久" and "火", which means that moxibustion is like long-lasting fire and has the function of warming and unblocking meridians. Similar to the natural water flow, the energy network stagnates in the cold state and can cause diseases over time. Traditional moxibustion releases energy by burning mugwort, which can stimulate acupoints and promote the flow of energy (qi) in meridians, so as to restore the normal balance of the body. Traditional moxibustion will produce a certain odor when burning the herb, which is generally believed to be harmless to the human body. Nowadays, there are also various kinds of smokeless moxibustion, whose specific efficacy is still controversial. Modern studies have found that moxibustion may affect the body by releasing infrared rays.

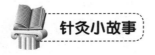

针灸小故事

1971 年，美国纽约时报记者 James 先生为准备尼克松访华事项提前来到中国。不幸的是，James 突发急性阑尾炎，在北京实施阑尾炎手术，并于次日晚，因腹部不适而接受针灸治疗。James 先生对于这项初次接受的治疗手段感到非常惊奇，并提到治疗之后"腹部压力明显减轻，之后这种不适没有复发"。回到美国之后，James 先生将这段神奇的经历发表在纽约时报上，引起了美国社会以及整个西方对针灸的关注，进而引发国际"针灸热"。

The story of Acupuncture:

In 1971, Mr. James, a reporter for the New York Times, came to China ahead of schedule to prepare for Nixon's visit to China. Unfortunately, James suddenly developed acute appendicitis and underwent am appendectomy in Beijing. The next day, he received acupuncture treatment for his post-surgical abdominal discomfort. Mr. James was very surprised by the treatment he received for the first time, and said that after the treatment, "the abdominal pressure was significantly reduced, and the discomfort did not recur". After returning to the United States, Mr. James published this amazing experience in the New York Times, which attracted the attention of American society and the entire Western world to acupuncture, which in turn triggering the international "acupuncture fever".

实践活动

1. 参观河南中医药大学第三附属医院针灸科。

2. 体验一次针灸治疗。

3. 与 3 ~ 5 位患者交流体会。

课后作业

对针灸治疗的体会，可以小组讨论。

Practical activities:

1. Visit the Acupuncture Department of the Third Affiliated Hospital of Henan University of Chinese Medicine.

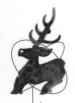

2. Experience acupuncture treatment once.

3. Communicate with 3-5 patients.

Homework

Group discussion—the experience of your acupuncture treatment.

二、拔罐

拔罐疗法利用各种材质的杯状器具（罐）对体表产生负压，使之吸附于体表或腧穴，使局部充血、瘀血，激发机体免疫系统，以达到治病和强身的目的。拔罐疗法拥有悠久的历史，世界各地如古埃及、古代欧洲、中东等地的传统医疗文献均有记载。

在中国，最早的拔罐疗法文字记载可以追溯到公元前 168 年。最初的拔罐器具以兽角为主，之后相继出现竹罐、陶制罐、玻璃罐、塑料罐

来华留学生中原中医药文化体验双语教程

A Chinese-English Course on Traditional Chinese Medicine for Foreign Students in China

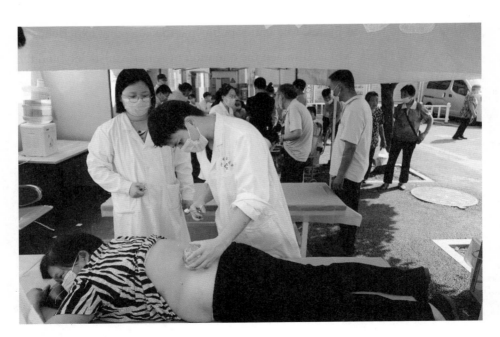

义诊现场（拔罐）

Volunteer Medical Treatment—Cupping

等。产生负压的方法包括水煮或药煮、燃火、真空抽气法等。其机理与热胀冷缩或者气体燃烧、排出有关。现代最常使用的为火罐和抽气罐。火罐使用酒精点火消耗罐内氧气形成负压，而抽气罐使用直接抽气的方式形成负压。目前拔罐疗法被大大丰富并扩展到内科、妇科、儿科、精神科等领域，通过排出内毒、疏通经络、激发经气达到治病强身的目的。现代临床一般常用于颈肩腰背疼痛、头痛、感冒、哮喘、咳嗽、痛经等。

现代研究认为拔罐疗法产生的负压使局部血流加速，毛细血管扩张，其内包含致病因素的血液溢出至组织间隙，激活免疫系统以清除毒素。拔罐配合刺血疗法则能加速毒素的排除，对顽固久病疗效更佳。同时，罐疗可以放松肌肉，减轻组织黏连，促进气血运行，对于各种运动之后的肌肉紧张、酸痛等有很好的帮助恢复的作用。

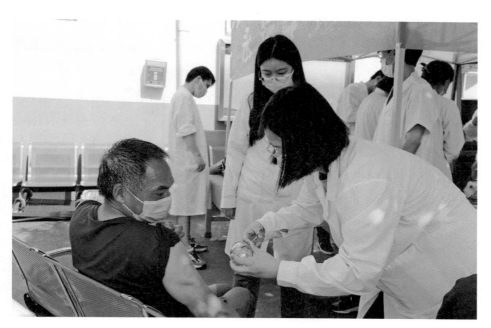

义诊现场（拔罐）

Volunteer Medical Treatment—Cupping

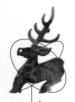

II. Cupping

Cupping therapy uses cup-shaped tools of various materials to generate negative pressure on the body surface, making the "cup" be adsorbed on the body surface. This technique can cause local congestion, and stimulate the body's immune system to achieve the purpose of curing diseases and strengthening the body. Cupping therapy has a long history and is recorded in traditional medical documents around the world, such as ancient Egypt, ancient Europe, and the Middle East.

In China, the earliest written records of cupping therapy that could be queried came from 168 BC. The original cupping utensils were mainly animal horns, followed by bamboo jars, ceramic jars, glass jars, plastic jars, and so on. As for the methods to generate negative pressure, there are ways like water boiling or Chinese medicine boiling, fire-burning, vacuum extraction and so on. The mechanism is related to thermal expansion and contraction, and gas combustion or discharge. The most commonly used cupping methods in modern times include fire-cupping and air extraction method. In fire-cupping, alcohol cotton balls are ignited to consume oxygen in the cup to create negative pressure; while in air extraction method, air in the cup is extracted directly for the creation of negative pressure. With the development of Chinese medicine, cupping therapy has been greatly enriched and expanded to many different fields, like internal medicine, gynecology, pediatrics, psychiatry, etc. By removing internal toxins and dredging the meridians, cupping therapy can strengthen the body and cure diseases. Nowadays, it's been widely used for neck/shoulder/back pain, headache, common cold, asthma, cough, dysmenorrhea, etc.

Modern research suggests that the negative pressure generated by cupping therapy can accelerate local blood flow, expand capillaries and also cause the blood containing pathogenic factors to leak into the interstitial spaces, which can activate the immune system to remove toxins. Cupping combined with lancet therapy can accelerate the elimination of toxins, and has a better effect on stubborn and chronic diseases. At the same time, cupping therapy can relax muscles, reduce tissue adhesion, promote the circulation of *qi* and blood, and help the recovery of muscle tension and soreness after various exercises.

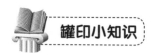 罐印小知识

拔罐疗法之后，局部因充血、瘀血，常常会留下罐口大小的印记，颜色或红或青或紫，偶有瘀斑或者水泡出现，被称为罐印或者罐斑，会随着时间自行消退，不留任何痕迹。罐印被认为是拔罐疗法能够起效的关键，不同颜色代表机体状况不同。例如，暗紫色代表体内有瘀血或者风寒，鲜红色代表有虚热。其印记不仅可以协助诊断机体的状态，其消退也代表着免疫系统激活以清除皮下组织废旧产物。拔罐过后，随着瘀血被清除，局部压力减轻，新鲜血液得以进入，带来新的活力，同时，罐印随之消除。

Some knowledge about cupping marks:

After the cupping therapy, marks of can-mouth size will show up, and the color may be red, blue, or purple, occasionally with bruises or blisters. These marks are called cupping marks or cupping spots and will fade spontaneously over time without leaving any traces. Cupping marks are considered to be the key for cupping therapy to be effective and different colors mean different body constitution. For example, dark purple usually means stagnation and cold, while bright red means internal heat. The marks can not only assist in diagnosing the state of the body, but the regression also represents the activation of the immune system, which can remove the waste products from the subcutaneous tissue. After cupping, as the congestion is cleared and the local pressure is reduced, fresh blood can enter the space and bring in new vitality. At the same time, the marks will fade away.

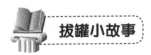
拔罐小故事

2016 年 8 月，31 岁的游泳明星菲尔普斯在里约热内卢奥运会上获得了他个人拿到的第 19 枚奥运金牌。人们在对他的成绩赞叹的同时，也被菲尔普斯身上暗红色的圆形印记吸引目光。"那是什么？"对于大部分美国观众来讲，这无疑是新奇的。菲尔普斯在采访中说道："过去两三年我一直都在拔火罐，我很喜欢，它对我的效果很明显，增加了我的灵活性，让我酸痛的肌肉可以放松。"菲利普斯在奥运会上为拔罐做了亲身宣传，引起美国社会对拔罐以及其他中医传统疗法的兴趣。

The story of Cupping:

In August 2016, the 31-year-old swimming star Phelps won his 19th personal Olympic gold medal at the Rio de Janeiro Olympics. While people were admiring his achievements, they were also attracted by the dark red circular marks on Phelps' back. "What is that?" For most American audiences, it was undoubtedly novel. Phelps said in the interview: "I have been under cupping therapy for the past two or three years. I like it very much. Its effect on me is obvious. It increases my flexibility and relaxes my sore muscles." Phelps personally promoted cupping therapy at the Olympics, which aroused the interest of cupping therapy and other traditional Chinese medicine therapies in American society.

实践活动

1. 参观河南中医药大学第三附属医院针灸科。

2. 体验一次拔罐治疗。

3. 与 3 ～ 5 位患者交流。

课后作业

1. 对拔罐治疗的体会，可以小组讨论。

2. 完成关于拔罐的测试题。

Practical activities

1. Visit the Acupuncture Department of the Third Affiliated Hospital of Henan University of Chinese Medicine.

2. Experience cupping treatment once.

3. Communicate with 3-5 patients.

Homework

1. The experience of cupping therapy can be discussed in groups.

2. Complete the test about cupping therapy.

125

三、推拿

推拿疗法是中医学不可分割的一部分，是在中医学理论的指导下，运用推拿手法或借助特定的推拿工具作用于体表的特定部位或穴位来治疗疾病的一种治疗方法，属于中医外治法范畴。

推拿的缘起可以追溯至史前时代。为了获得必要的生活资料，我们的祖先逐渐掌握了攀爬、开荒、跋涉、打猎等技能，再加上恶劣的自然环境，身体的外伤出血在所难免。他们出于本能的自我治疗意识，自然而然地通过按压达到止血的目的、摩病患以消肿，因而产生了推拿早期比较简单的按法和摩法。随着日积月累、口口相传，一些原始的推拿手法得以总结和传承，历经夏、商、周三代的培育，至秦汉时期，推拿从理论到实践已具雏形。推拿发展至明代，又出现了一个新的分支——小儿推拿

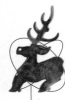

疗法。

随着社会的进步，人们更加深刻认识到天然药物疗法和非药物疗法的优越性。推拿这一简便、高效、无毒、无副作用、不药而愈的治疗方法越来越为人们所青睐，引起国际医务界的重视；中国推拿与国外进行了广泛的交流，中国推拿学者出国讲学、医疗，赢得了国外的好评；同时，不少国家和地区的推拿专业人员也来中国学习中医推拿，且人员日益增多。

With the progress of society, people are more deeply aware of the advantages of natural drug therapy and non drug therapy. Massage therapy Tuina, a traditional simple, efficient, non-toxic, non side effect and non drug treatment method, is more and more favored by people, which has attracted the attention of the international medical community. Chinese Massage Therapy Tuina has carried out extensive exchanges with foreign countries, and won the praise of foreign countries; at the same time, more and more people come to China to study Chinese Massage Therapy Tuina.

Ⅲ. Tuina Therapy

Tuina Therapy is an inseparable part of traditional Chinese medicine. It is a kind of treatment method to treat diseases by using massage techniques or using certain massage tools to act on specific parts or acupoints on the body surface under the guidance of traditional Chinese medicine theory. It belongs to the category of external treatment of traditional Chinese medicine.

The origin of Massage Therapy can be traced back to prehistoric times. In order to obtain the necessary means of living, climbing, reclaiming wasteland, trekking and hunting were the daily behaviors of the ancestors, and the harsh natural environment became a problem they often had to face and deal with. As a result, body trauma and bleeding were inevitable. Out of the human instinct of self-treatment, pressing to stop bleeding and rubbing to reduce swelling were the natural behaviors in dealing with injuries. This resulted in the relatively simple pressing method and rubbing method in the early stage of Massage Therapy. With the accumulation of time, some primitive massage techniques can be summarized and inherited. After the cultivation of Xia, Shang and Zhou dynasties, Massage Therapy has taken shape from theory to practice in Qin and Han dynasties. In the Ming Dynasty, a new branch of Massage Therapy appeared—Pediatric Massage Therapy.

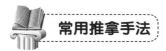

常用推拿手法

擦法：在受术部位做单向直线来回摩擦运动的手法，称为擦法。根据着力部位的不同，可分为小鱼际擦法、大鱼际擦法、掌擦法等。

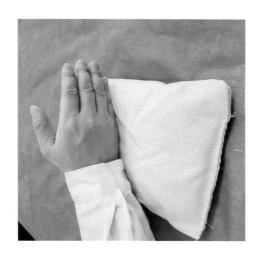

小鱼际擦法
Thenar rubbing method

Commonly used Massage techniques:

Rubbing method: Ca Fa (Rubbing method): a one-way straight back and forth rubbing movement on the subject site, According to the different parts of the force, it can be divided into small thenar rubbing method, large thenar rubbing method, palm rubbing method and so on.

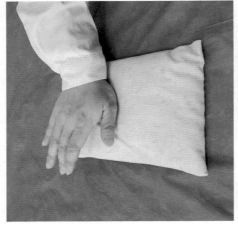

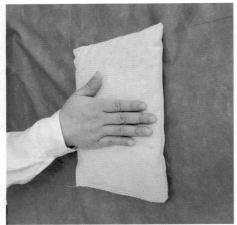

大鱼际擦法

Large thenar rubbing method

掌擦法

Palm rubbing method

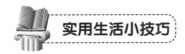

实用生活小技巧

1. 横擦腰骶部治疗痛经

痛经是女性常见的妇科症状之一，主要表现为经期前后或月经期出现下腹痉挛性疼痛、坠胀、伴腰酸或其他全身不适，严重者影响日常生活和工作。在生活工作中我们经常可以遇到痛经的女性，推拿可有效缓解痛经。

Practical tips

1. Treatment of dysmenorrhea by applying Ca Fa (backward-forward rubbing method) horizontally on the lumbosacral region

Dysmenorrhea is one of the most common gynecological symptoms among women. It is mainly manifested as spasmodic pain in the lower abdomen, distension, backache or other systemic discomfort before and after menstruation or during menstruation, which may seriously affect daily life

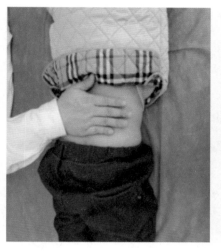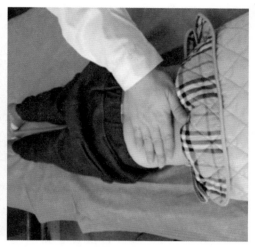

横擦腰骶部

Treatment of dysmenorrhea by applying Ca Fa (backward-forward rubbing method) horizontally on the lumbosacral region

and work. In life and work, we often meet women with dysmenorrhea, and massage therapy tuina can effectively relieve dysmenorrhea.

2. 擦鼻翼两侧治疗鼻炎

鼻炎是临床常见的疾病之一，其患病率也逐年增加。鼻炎主要表现为鼻塞、流涕、打喷嚏，还会出现头晕、头痛、嗅觉降低，严重的可以出现记忆力减退等，对人体健康及正常生活带来很大困扰。推拿治疗鼻炎有立竿见影的优势。

2. Treatment of Rhinitis by wiping both sides of nasal alar

Rhinitis is one of the common clinical diseases, and its prevalence rate is increasing year by year. Rhinitis is mainly manifested as nasal congestion, runny nose, sneezing, dizziness, headache, decreased sense of smell, serious memory loss, etc., which brings great trouble to human health and normal life. Massage treatment of rhinitis has an immediate advantage.

实践活动

1. 到推拿科门诊参观。

2. 根据身体状况体验推拿疗法。

Practical Activities:

1. Visit the Massage Therapy Department.

2. Experience Massage Therapy Therapy according to personal physical condition.

四、刮痧

刮痧是用刮痧器具反复刮拭体表，使之发红，出现片状或块状的青紫瘀斑或瘀点，以治疗或预防疾病的一种自然疗法。

刮痧疗法起源于远古时代。据文献记载，上古之人病时，常常本能地用手或拾起石块摩刮患部或体表某一部位，有时竟获病痛缓解或痊愈的奇效，这种偶然获得的疗效经反复多次实践运用，再经人们口耳相传，不断总结积累，逐渐形成一种有效的治疗方法。关于刮痧疗法最早的文字记载见于湖南长沙马王堆汉墓出土的春秋战国时期的古老帛书《五十二病方》。该书介绍了运用砭石直接在皮表刮拭，或用砭石作为热熨，以治疗疾病。

随着刮痧疗法的发展，刮痧器具进一步丰富多样，可分为民间使用与专业使用两类。民间使用的刮痧器具多为因地制宜、简便易寻者，如玉石、牛角、汤匙、小碗、杯、盘、硬币等，种类繁多；专业使用者较为精致，目前多以牛角制品为主。

现代刮痧疗法集局部按摩、穴位刺激和药物治疗为一体，治疗范围扩展到内科、外科、伤科、妇科、儿科、眼科、养颜美容、减肥保健等领域，通过疏通经络、激发经气达到治病保健、美容减肥的目的。其施术作用大致可分为提高机体免疫力和治疗疾病两大类。

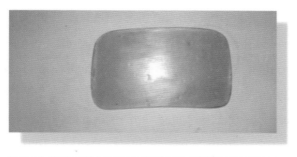

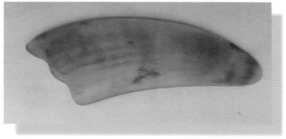

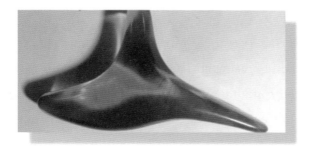

各种类型的刮痧器具
Various types of scraping implements

Ⅳ. The Gua Sha Treatment

Guasha therapy is a kind of natural therapy to treat or prevent diseases by repeatedly scraping the body surface with scraping tools to make it red and appear pieces of purple ecchymosis or ecchymosis.

Guasha therapy originated in ancient times. According to literature, when people were sick, they often instinctively used their hands or picked up stones

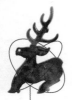
to rub and scrape, hit the affected part or a certain part of the body surface, and sometimes achieved the miraculous effect of pain relief or recovery. This kind of accidental curative effect has been used repeatedly, and then passed on, and gradually formed an effective treatment method. The earliest written record of the Gua Sha Treatment can be found in the silk manuscript *Fifty-two Diseases Prescription* unearthed from Mawangdui Han Dynasty Tomb of the Spring and Autumn and Warring States periods in Changsha, Hunan Province .

With the development of the Gua Sha Treatment, Gua Sha apparatus is more abundant and diverse, which can be divided into two types: folk use and professional use. Most of the scraping instruments used by people are simple and easy to find according to local conditions, such as jade, ox horn, spoon, small bowl, cup, plate, coin, etc; the professional scraping instruments, are mostly horn products.

Modern Gua Sha Treatment integrates local massage therapy, acupoint stimulation and drug treatment. The scope of treatment is extended to internal medicine, surgery, traumatology, gynecology, pediatrics, ophthalmology, beauty, weight loss and health care. By dredging the meridians and stimulating the meridians, it can achieve the purpose of disease treatment, health care, beauty and weight loss. It can be divided into two categories: improving immunity and treating diseases.

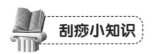

刮痧刺激后皮肤表面会出现红、紫、黑斑或小点状紫红色疹子，并伴有不同程度的热痛感等现象，称为"出痧"。出痧的过程是一种血管扩张至毛细血管破裂、血流外溢、皮肤局部形成血斑的现象，能加强局部的新陈代谢，有消炎的作用，是刮痧后出现的正常反应，一般不需作

特殊处理。

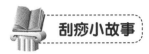

刮痧小故事

2001 年上映的电影《刮痧》以中医刮痧疗法产生误会为主线，讲述了华人在国外由于中西方文化的冲突而陷入种种困境：男主人公五岁的丹尼斯闹肚发烧，在家的爷爷因为看不懂药品上的英文说明，便用中国民间流传的刮痧疗法给丹尼斯治病，刮痧留下的痧痕意外成为男主人公虐待孩子的证据……随着中外文化交流的加深，尤其是里约奥运会，美国游泳名将菲尔普斯身上那一个又一个的罐印，让更多外国人通过各式各样的途径、渠道来了解中国，引起国际社会对中医传统外治疗法的兴趣。

Knowledge of the Gua Sha Treatment

After Gua Sha stimulation, there will be red, purple, dark spots or small purple-red rashes on the skin surface, accompanied by different sensations like heat and pain, which is called "Chu Sha". The process of "Chu Sha" is a phenomenon in which blood vessels expand and capillary rupture, causing blood spots on the skin. It can speed up local metabolism and has anti-inflammatory effects. It is a normal reaction that appears after Gua Sha. Generally, no special treatment is required.

Stories about the Gua Sha Treatment

The film *The Gua Sha Treatment* "scraping" released in 2001 focuses on the misunderstanding of traditional Chinese medicine scraping therapy. It tells the story of Chinese people falling into various difficulties due to the conflict between Chinese and Western cultures abroad: Five-year-old Dennis has a fever and suffers from diarrhoea , and his grandfather at home uses the Chinese Gua Sha Treatment to treat Dennis because he can't understand the English words on the medicine. The scraping marks left by scraping have unexpectedly

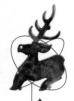

become evidence of the grandfather's abuse of children... With the deepening of cultural exchanges between China and foreign countries, especially in the Rio Olympic Games, the cupping marks on the famous American swimmer Phelps have aroused the interest of the international community in the traditional external treatment of traditional Chinese medicine.

实践活动

1. 到河南中医药大学第三附属医院推拿科门诊参观。

2. 根据身体状况体验刮痧疗法。

Practical Activities:

1. Visit the Massage Therapy Department of the Third Affiliated Hospital of Henan University of Traditional Chinese Medicine.

2. Experience the Gua Sha Treatment according to personal physical condition.

134

第四节　中医气功养生文化实践

一、太极拳

太极拳是中国特有的养生功法，是中国传统文化之一，于 2020 年 12 月 17 日被联合国教科文组织（UNESCO）正式列入"人类非物质文化遗产代表作名录"，目前在世界上的受众超过 4 亿人。太极拳起源的说法不一，现多数认为其起源于河南省温县陈家沟，是陈王廷于明末清初（17 世纪中叶）结合传统儒、道哲学与中医经络学说，以及古代导引、吐纳之术创立的。后经杨露缠、吴鉴泉、武禹襄、孙禄堂等传承发展，衍生出杨氏、武氏、孙氏等不同派系，可用于强身健体，也可用于攻防竞技，老少皆宜。

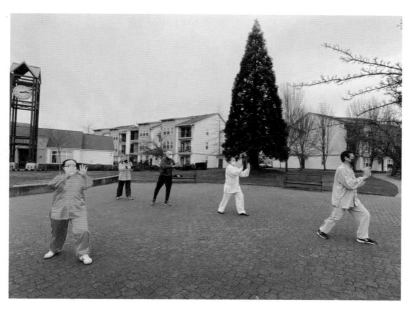

太极拳（1）

Tai Chi Quan (1)

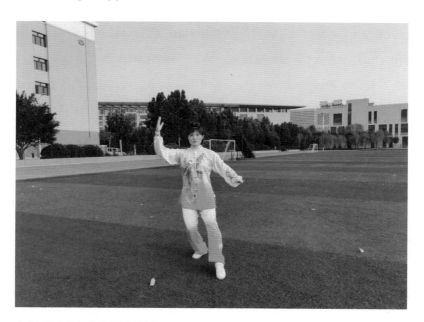

太极拳（2）（白鹤亮翅）

Tai Chi—White Stork Stretching Wings

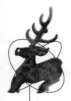

现代流行的太极多以养生保健为目的。与西方运动健身相比，太极内敛含蓄，以"天人合一""中正自然"为理念，动作柔和，缓急相间，行云流水。其具体动作讲究"气沉丹田（位于小腹部）"，心身合一，以腰背和脊柱为轴，全身各个部位协调运动。

Section IV Experience and Practice of Traditional Chinese Medicine Qigong Health Preservation

Ⅰ. Tai Chi Quan

Taiji Quan is a unique health-preserving exercise in China and one part of the traditional Chinese culture. On December 17, 2020, it was officially included in the "Representative List of the Intangible Cultural Heritage of Humanity" by UNESCO. There are more than 400 million people practicing Taiji Quan in the world. Although there are different opinions on the origin of Taiji Quan, most people believe that it originated in Chenjiagou, Wenxian County, Henan Province, where Chen Wangting created this activity in the late Ming and early Qing dynasties (about mid 17th century) by combining traditional Confucian culture, Taoist philosophy, and the ancient techniques of moving and breathing with the meridian theory of traditional Chinese medicine. Later on, different factions were derived through the inheritance and development of Taiji Quan by Yang Luchan, Wu Jianquan, Sun Lutang, etc. Taiji Quan is suitable for all ages and can be used for physical fitness, as well as offensive and defensive competitions.

Taiji Quan in modern times mostly aims at health preservation. Compared with Western sports and fitness, Taiji Quan is introverted and reserved. It is based on the concept of "Harmony between Man and Nature" and "Balance

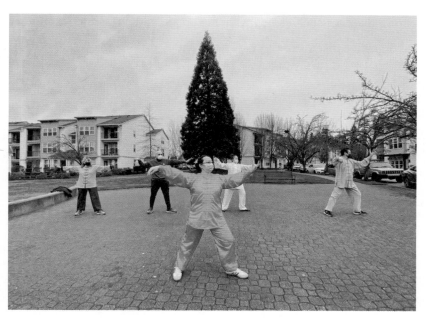

太极拳 (3)
Taiji Quan (3)

and Nature". Its movements are soft, slow and deliberate. The specific action emphasizes "the Qi sinks into the pubic region (located in the lower abdomen)" and "Mind-Body Unity", with the waist and spine acting as the axis to coordinate the movement of all parts of the body.

　　与一般运动相比，太极拳因其注重"抱神守一"而具有冥想的特点，又因其参考中医经络理论并注重气机流畅而具有激活经络系统、通气活血的作用，故而不仅可以强身健体，提升免疫力，而且对于神经衰弱、焦虑、抑郁、呼吸系统、消化系统等慢性病均有很好的改善效果。

Compared with general exercises, Taiji Quan has the characteristics of meditation because of its emphasis on "holding the spirit and keeping one". It also has the function of activating the meridian system and moving Qi and blood because of its reference to the TCM meridian theory. Therefore, it can not only strengthen the body, boost the immune system, but also has a good

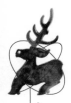

effect on curing diseases such as neurasthenia, anxiety, depression, respiratory diseases and digestive diseases.

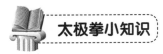

太极拳小知识

虽然太极有不同流派，但是其区别仅限于动作构成，而基本理念仍然相同。以陈氏太极为例，陈王廷拥有武学基础，故而其创立的太极具有纵跳、震足等高难度动作。而杨氏太极则删改了高难度动作，以满足一般练拳人的需要。其他的太极流派同样各有特点，与其创始人的背景、经历相关。1956年，国家体育总局组织太极拳专家从杨氏太极拳中汲取精华，形成二十四式简化太极拳，因其内容精炼、动作规范而广泛流行。

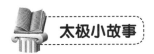

太极小故事

陈王廷自幼天资聪慧，勤奋好学，文武双全。然而，在明末清初动荡的环境中，陈王廷报国无门。于是他返乡归隐，一边耕种养家，一边研究拳法。陈玉廷自幼便练习家传武学，在隐居期间，他搜集、整理民间武术，融诸家之长，除太极拳外，他还传授下来长拳、刀、剑、棍等器械功法。

Some knowledge about Tai Chi Quan:

Although there are different Taiji Quan genres, the differences are limited to the composition of their actions, and the basic idea remains the same. Take Chen's Taiji Quan for example, Chen Wangting has the foundation of martial arts, so his style has many complicated and difficult movements such as vertical jump and foot shaking. The Yang style has deleted and changed the difficult movements to meet the needs of general practitioners. Other

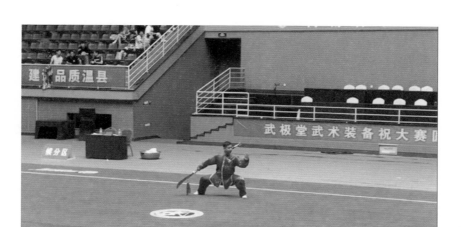

太极器械比赛

Equipment Competition of Tai Chi

Taiji Quan genres also have their own characteristics, which are related to the background and experience of their founders. In 1956, the State Sports General Administration gathered Taiji Quan experts to draw the essence from Yang's Taiji Quan and formed a twenty-four simplified Taiji Quan, which has been widely popular because of its refined content and standardized movements.

The story of Taiji Quan:

Chen Wangting was talented, hardworking, and eager to learn since childhood. However, in the turbulent society environment in the late Ming and early Qing dynasties, he could not find a way to serve the country. As a result, he returned to his hometown and studied martial arts while farming to support his family. Chen Wangting has been practicing his family martial arts since he was a child. During his seclusion, he collected and organized folk martial arts, and integrated the strengths of various families. In addition to Taiji Quan, he also handed down other equipment exercises, such as blades, swords, sticks, etc.

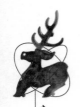
实践活动

1. 参观太极拳表演。

2. 学习一个简单太极动作。

课后作业

撰写一篇对于太极的体验感想短文。

Practical activities

1. Visit the performance of Taiji Quan.

2. Learn a simple Taiji Quan movement.

Homework

Write a short essay about Taiji Quan experience.

二、八段锦

八段锦也是中国传统养生功法之一，由八个动作构成。锦是古代上等丝织品，用多种不同颜色编织而成，有柔和优美之意，以作为此功法的美称。关于八段锦最早的文字记载出现于晋朝，而其具体为何人、何时所创尚无定论。因其简单易学，自宋朝时代起便广泛流传，至今已衍生出多个不同的流派。根据练功时站坐的不同，分为动式八段锦（站式）与静式八段锦（坐式）。而站式又可分为南北两派，其中北派动作繁杂、难度大，而南派动作柔和简单，较北派流传广。现行流传的八段锦是中国国家体育总局健身气功管理中心以南派八段锦为蓝图组织改编的。

八段锦由八个动作构成，其功用各异：

第一式：双手托天理三焦。此动作两手上举如将天托起，主要用于调理心肺，疏通三焦经和心包经，促进血液循环，同时可以调整脊柱两侧的肌肉、自律神经等。

第二式：左右开工似射雕。此动作可以扩张胸部，利于心肺，疏通肺经，同时可以锻炼肩背部、手臂肌肉。

第三式：调理脾胃需单举。主要用于调理脾胃，对于消化系统有很好的作用。

第四式：五劳七伤往后瞧。可强健肺脏，同时通过扭转可激活背部经络，尤其是脊柱两边的内脏神经。

第五式：摇头摆尾去心火。大幅度的动作，使五脏六腑得到内在按摩，使胸腹的郁火得以消除，从而起到去心火的作用。

第六式：双手攀足固肾腰。此动作通过伸展背腰部筋膜，可缓解腰痛，同时可强固肾脏。

第七式：攒拳怒目增气力。此动作运动上肢、胁肋部以及眼部，可梳理肝气，强筋养目。

第八式：背后七颠百病消。利用颠足使得脊柱轻微抖动，疏通气血，帮助脊柱周围组织的液体交换。

与太极拳相比，八段锦动作同样注重心身合一，然而其动作更为简单，讲究柔和缓慢，不具有技击防身的用途，单纯用于强身健体。现代研究发现，八段锦对于各种慢性疾患，如慢性阻塞性肺疾病、2型糖尿病、焦虑、

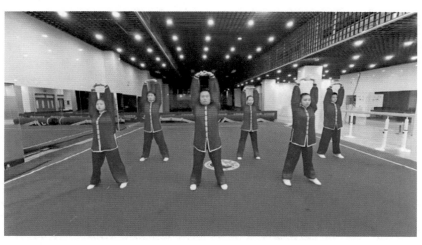

八段锦第一式
Eight Trigrams Boxing

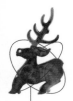

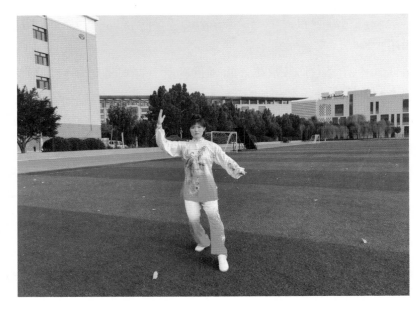

八段锦第二式
Baduan Jin-The second posture

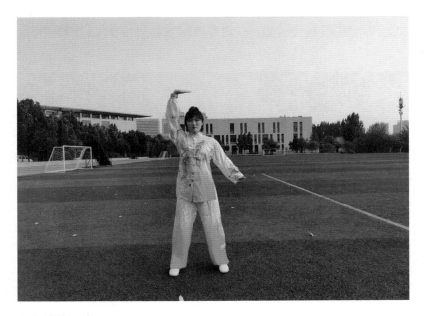

八段锦第三式
Baduan Jin-The Third posture

来华留学生中原中医药文化体验双语教程

A Chinese-English Course on Traditional Chinese Medicine for Foreign Students in China

抑郁、冠心病等，均有很好的辅助效果。

‖. Baduan Jin

Eight Trigrams Boxing (Baduan Jin) is also one of the traditional Chinese health-preserving exercises. "Baduan" means this exercise consists of eight movements. "Jin" is an ancient fine silk fabric, woven with a variety of different colors and has a soft and graceful meaning. The earliest written records about Baduan Jin appeared in the Jin Dynasty, but it is still unclear by whom and when it was created. Because of its simplicity and ease of learning, it has been widely spread since the Song Dynasty, and many different genres have been derived so far. According to the differences of standing or sitting during practice, it is divided into dynamic Baduan Jin (standing) and static Baduan Jin (sitting). The standing style can be divided into two groups: the north style and the south style. The movements of the north style are complicated and difficult, while of the south style are soft and simple, hence the south one is more popular. The current widely popular Baduan Jin is an adaptation based on the south style by the Health Qigong Management Center of the State Sports General Administration.

Baduan Jin consists of eight movements, each of which has different functions:

The first movement: Two hands supporting the sky to regulate Sanjiao

This posture is mainly used to regulate the heart and lungs, dredge the triple burner meridian and pericardium meridian, promote blood circulation, and adjust the muscles on both sides of the spine, as well as autonomic nerves.

The second posture: Drawing bows to the left and right

This posture can expand the chest, help the heart and lungs, clear the lung meridian, and exercise the shoulder, back, and arm muscles.

The third posture: Single hand pushing up to regulate the spleen

This posture is mainly used to regulate the spleen and stomach, and has a good effect on the digestive system.

The fourth posture: Turning head to look back

This posture can strengthen the lung and activate the meridians and the visceral nerves on both sides of the spine by twisting the body.

The fifth posture: Moving head and tailbone to clear heart fire

Through large-scale movements, the organs can get a internal massage, so that the depression of the chest and abdomen can be eliminated, which helps to clear the heart fire.

The sixth posture: Both hands reaching the ground to strengthen the kidney

This posture can stretch the back and waist fascia to relieve low back pain and also strengthen the kidneys.

The seventh posture: Clenching the fists and glaring fiercely to be stronger.

This movement exercises the upper limbs, flank and eyes. It can comb the liver qi, strengthen the muscles and nourish the eyes.

The eighth posture: Bouncing on the toes to relieve various issues.

The use of foot trembling makes the spine slightly shake, moving qi and blood, and helping the fluid exchange of the tissues around the spine.

Similar to Taiji Quan, Baduan Jin also pays attention to the unity of mind and body, but its movements are simpler, gentler and slower, without the purpose of attack or defense. They are only used for physical fitness. Modern studies have found that Baduan Jin has a good auxiliary effect on various chronic diseases, such as chronic obstructive pulmonary disease, type II diabetes, anxiety, depression, and coronary heart disease, etc.

实践活动

1. 参观八段锦表演。

2. 选择学习一个八段锦动作。

课后作业

根据自己的体验比较八段锦与太极拳的异同。

Practical activities

1. Visit the performance of Baduan Jin.

2. Choose to learn a Baduan Jin movement.

Homework

Compare the similarities and differences between Baduan Jin and Taiji Quan based on your own experience.

三、五禽戏

五禽戏是东汉末年华佗（145–208）模仿五种飞禽走兽（虎、鹿、熊、猿、鸟）的动作形态而创作的导引术，具有强身健体的效果，其动作简单有趣，老少皆宜。2011 年五禽戏被纳入中国国家级非物质文化遗产项目。

与其他健身气功类似，五禽戏发展至今形成了不同的流派。华佗故里流行的主要是董氏和刘氏，其中董氏动作古朴典雅，而刘氏认为五禽戏亦属武术范畴，除徒手套路外还有器械套路。现行国家体育总局发布的五禽戏是按照虎、鹿、熊、猿、鸟的顺序，每戏 2 个动作，共 10 个动作，以模仿动物的动作、形态。每戏主要针对不同器官以及不同肢体部位。

虎戏主要锻炼肝脏，通过手型以及眼神模仿虎以达到养肝、舒筋、明目的效果。

鹿戏主要锻炼肾脏，其动作包含运转尾闾，刺激肾脏以及督脉，以改善生殖系统功能。

熊戏主要锻炼脾胃，通过模仿熊晃动身体，挤压按摩脾胃，调理中焦。

猿戏主要锻炼心脏，通过模仿猿猴摘果而后回头探看的动作，上肢大幅度运动，以及收腋以刺激心经，挤压按摩胸廓以增强心脏功能。

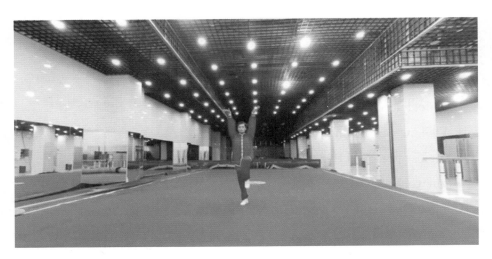

五禽戏之虎戏
The tiger posture

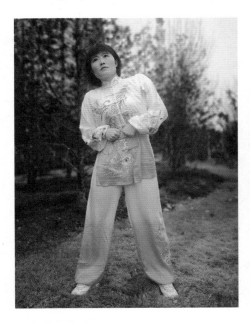

五禽戏之熊戏
Five Animal Boxing

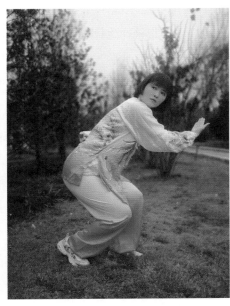

五禽戏之猿戏
Wuqin XI-The ape posture

鸟戏主要锻炼肺部功能，通过模仿鸟类开合翅膀，以疏通肺部经气。

现代研究发现，五禽戏对于循环系统、呼吸系统、免疫系统、运动骨骼系统以及心理健康方面均有很好的辅助效果。

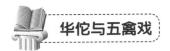
华佗与五禽戏

华佗是东汉末年著名的医学家，从少时便钻研医术，游历各地，声誉颇著。相传最早的麻醉剂"麻沸

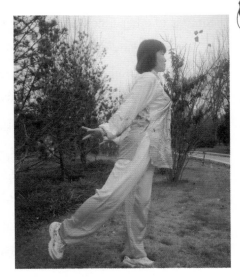
五禽戏之鸟戏
Wuqin Xi-The bird posture

147

散"即为华佗所创。华佗认为人体需要经常运动但是不能过量。适量的运动能够增强消化系统，促进血液流通，从而起到防治疾病的效果。受传统中医的"天人合一"思想及五行理论的启发，华佗通过观察模仿自然界生物的运动而创制五禽戏。其中虎之勇猛对应肝，鹿之安舒对应肾，熊之沉稳对应脾，猿之灵巧对应心，鸟之敏捷对应肺。相传其弟子吴璞练习五禽戏，活到90多岁，仍然耳聪目明，牙齿完好。

Ⅲ. Wuqin Xi (Five Animal Boxing)

Wuqin Xi was created by Hua Tuo (145-208) in the late eastern Han Dynasty. He imitated the movements of five kinds of animals, including the tiger, the deer, the bear, the ape and the bird, to strengthen the body. The movements of Wuqin Xi are simple and interesting, which make the exercise suitable for all ages. In 2011, it was included in China's National Intangible Cultural Heritage Project.

Similar to other fitness qigong exercises, Wuqin Xi has different schools. In Hua Tuo's hometown, the most popular ones are Dong's style and Liu's style. Among them, Dong's movements are simple and elegant, while Liu's style is more similar to martial arts and also has movements with equipments. The current Wuqin Xi issued by the National General Administration of Sports follows the order of tiger, deer, bear, ape, and bird, with two actions in each play and a total of ten actions to imitate the actions and forms of animals. Each posture targets at different organs and different body parts.

The tiger posture mainly exercises the liver, and its movements can relax the tendons and improve the eyesight. The movements imitate the tiger's action through the shape of the hands and the spirit in the eyes.

The deer posture mainly exercises the kidney. Its actions include running the tail, stimulating the kidney and governor channel to improve the function of the reproductive system.

The bear posture mainly exercises the spleen and stomach by imitating the bear shaking the body to squeeze and massage the spleen and stomach.

The ape posture mainly exercises the heart by imitating the ape's action of picking fruits from the tree and then looking back to squeeze and massage the chest, thus stimulating the heart meridian and enhancing the heart function.

The bird posture mainly exercises the lung function by imitating the opening and closing of birds' wings to dredge the lung meridian.

Modern research has found that Wuqin Xi has a good auxiliary effect on the circulatory system, the respiratory system, the immune system, the musculoskeletal system, and mental health.

Hua Tuo and Wuqin Xi:

Hua Tuo was a famous traditional Chinese medicine doctor in the late

Eastern Han Dynasty. He studied medicine from a very young age and traveled all over the country to treat patients. It is said that the earliest anesthetic "Mafei San" was created by him. Hua Tuo believed that the human body needs to exercise regularly, but not excessively. Moderate exercise can enhance the digestive system, promote blood circulation, thereby preventing and treating diseases. Based on the TCM concept of "harmony between man and nature" and the theory of five elements, Hua Tuo created Wuqin Xi by observing and imitating the movement of natural creatures. Among them, the bravery of tiger corresponds to the liver, the ease of deer corresponds to the kidney, the calmness of bear corresponds to the spleen, the dexterity of ape corresponds to the heart, and the agility of bird corresponds to the lung. It is said that Wu Pu, his disciple, practiced Wuqin Xi and lived to be over 90 years old. Regardless of his age, his eyes and ears were still good and his teeth were intact.

实践活动

1. 参观五禽戏表演。

2. 选择学习一个五禽戏动作。

课后作业

根据自己的体验比较八段锦、太极拳与五禽戏的异同。

Practical activities

1. Visit the performance of Wuqin Xi.

2. Choose to learn a movement action of Wuqin Xi.

Homework

Compare Baduan Jin, Tai Chi Quan and Wuqin Xi according to your own experience.

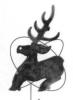
四、易筋经

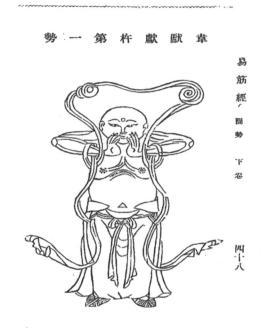

《易筋经》：韦陀献杵第一势
Yijin Jing: The first posture

易筋经与其他中国特色健身气功（导引术）一样，具有强健身体、养生保健、防治疾病、延缓衰老的功效。"易"有"变易"之意，"筋"即为肌肉筋膜（经络），"易筋"在此有强健筋骨、改变体质之意，"经"指"经典"。《易筋经》成书年代以及作者未有定论，一般认为成书于明清时代，对其作者的推论涉及道、释、医、武四家。

易筋经讲究精神放松，心身合一，呼吸自然，刚柔相济。传统易筋经包含内经和外经，各有十二势动作，以达到内壮和外壮的效果。内经多采用静止性发力，现行的健身气功易筋经以外壮为主，讲究"静虑凝神，通身不必用力，只须使其气贯两手"，个别动作难度较大，对肌肉力量的增强作用优于八段锦、五禽戏。

现代研究发现易筋经能够辅助治疗改善颈椎病、上交叉综合征、退行性膝关节炎、原发性纤维肌痛综合征以及预防老年人衰老性肌萎缩等。

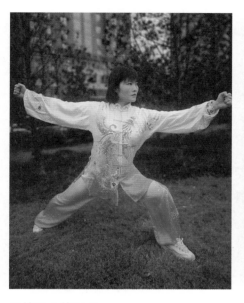

易筋经之第五式

Yijin Jing-The fifth posture

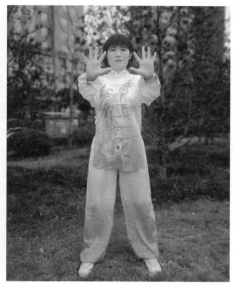

易筋经之第六式

Yijin Jing-The sixth posture

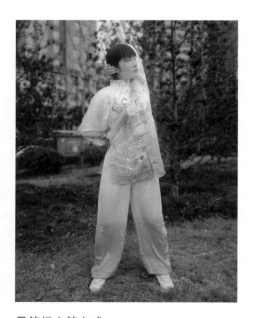

易筋经之第七式

Yijin Jing-The seventh posture

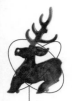
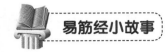 易筋经小故事

在现代，提到易筋经，大多数人会联想到少林寺僧侣。虽然实际考证发现其起源于少林达摩的说法并无文献支持，但是在易筋经的流传中，少林僧侣起到了重要的作用。由于禅宗的僧侣在静修时大多久坐，日久则导致气血流通不畅，进而气血枯萎，身体羸弱，故而需要导引术活动筋骨，使气血得以流通。少林寺僧侣在此过程中不断对其内容进行修改完善，而成为一种特殊的习武健身方式。

Ⅳ. Yijin Jing

Yijin Jing (Muscle-bone Tendon-muscle Strengthening Exercise), just like other traditional Chinese qigong exercises, has the functions of strengthening the body, maintaining good health, preventing diseases, and delaying aging. "Yi" means "changing", and "Jin" means muscle fascia (meridians). "Yijin" means strengthening muscles and bones and changing the constitution. "Jing" means "classic". *Yijin Jing* is a monograph on this qigong exercise. There's controversial opinions on its author and completion time. It is generally believed that the book was written in the Ming and Qing dynasties. The inference about its author involves four schools: Taoism, Buddhism, Chinese medicine, and martial arts.

Yijin Jing emphasizes relaxation of the spirit, unity of mind and body, natural breathing, and harmony between rigidity and softness. The traditional Yijin Jing contained inner and outer classics, each of which included twelve movements to achieve the effect of inner and outer strengthening. The current fitness Qigong Yijin Jing focuses on external strengthening, which stresses that one should "meditate and concentrate, and make the qi run through both hands without exerting force". Some movements are a little difficult, but the enhancement effect on muscle strength is better than Baduan Jin and Wuqin Xi.

Modern studies have found that Yijin Jing can assist in the treatment of cervical spondylosis, superior cruciate syndrome, degenerative knee arthritis, primary fibromyalgia syndrome, and so on. It is also believed to benefit the prevention of senile muscular atrophy in the elderly.

The story of Yijin Jing:

In modern times, when it comes to Yijin Jing, most people will associate it with Shaolin monks. Although there is no literature support for the claim that it originated from Shaolin Bodhidharma, Shaolin monks played an important role in the spread of Yijin Jing. The monks spent a lot of time sitting in meditation, which led to poor circulation of Qi and blood, and further caused Qi and blood withered, as well as the body weakened. Thus, they needed to guide the movement of muscles and bones to enhance the circulation of Qi and blood. In this process, the monks of Shaolin Temple constantly modified and perfected the content of Yijin Jing, which became a special way of practicing martial arts.

153

实践活动

1. 参观易筋经表演。

2. 选择学习一个易筋经动作。

课后作业

根据自己的体验比较易筋经与八段锦、太极拳、五禽戏的异同。

Practical activities

1. Visit the performance of Yijin Jing.

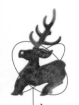

2. Choose to learn one Yijin Jing movement.

Homework

According to your own experience, compare the similarities and differences between Yijin Jing, Baduan Jin, Tai Chi Quan, and Wuqin Xi.

第五节　中医食疗

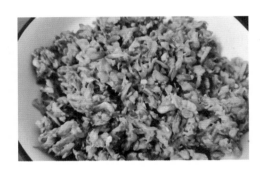

菜肴
Dishes

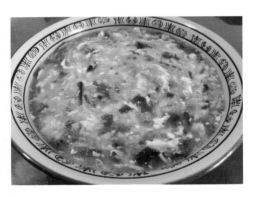

养生粥
Porridge

食疗，即用饮食治疗疾病，是根据患者病情需要，在中医理论指导下，通过合理的烹调加工，选择性地食用各种不同性能、具有一定治疗作用的食物，以作用到不同的脏器，从而达到调理和治愈疾病的目的。

食疗是中医药学重要组成部分，有悠久的历史。早在2 500年前的春秋战国时期，就有了食疗的分科。中国最早的医学专著《黄帝内经》即有"药以祛之，食以随之，谷肉果菜，食养尽之"的记载，它可以说是食物疗法最早的理论基础。即使在现代，食疗也仍然是疾病综合治疗中不可或缺的一部分。

食疗的种类丰富多样，主要包括菜肴、养生粥、养生汤羹、糖、蜜饯、药茶、药酒等。

中医食疗不仅在中国有悠久历史，而且对外国也有影响。随着人们

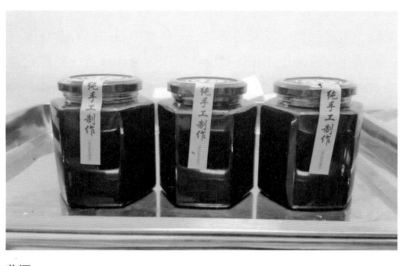

药酒

Medicinal liquor

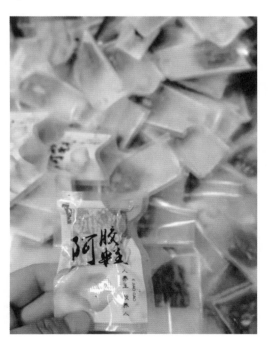

糕点

Pastry

155

生活水平不断提高，亚健康人群的不断增加，中西医结合食疗的产生与发展是社会需求和历史发展的必然。近年来中西医结合食疗逐步迈向整体化、精确化、预防优先化、社会化、国际化和经济效益优化，而且越来越受到医学界的重视。

Section Ⅴ　Dietotherapy of the Traditional Chinese Medicine

Dietotherapy, that is to treat diseases with diet, is to selectively eat various foods with different properties and certain therapeutic effects according to the needs of patients under the guidance of traditional Chinese medicine theory, so as to achieve the purpose of conditioning and curing diseases.

Dietotherapy is an important part of the treasure of Chinese medicine and has a long history. As early as 2,500 years ago in the Spring and Autumn Period and the Warring States Period, there was a division of dietotherapy. The earliest medical monograph *Huangdi Neijing* (*Huangdi's Internal Classic*) in China has the record that "medicine dispels it, food follows it, grain, meat, fruits and vegetables, eat and nourish it". It can be said to be the earliest theoretical basis of food therapy. Even in modern times, dietotherapy is still an indispensable part of comprehensive treatment of diseases.

There are various types of dietotherapy, mainly including dishes, porridge, soup, therapeutic sugar, preserves, medicinal tea, pastry and medicinal liquor.

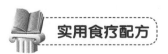
实用食疗配方

1. 生姜红糖水

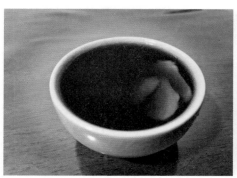

生姜红糖水

Ginger brown sugar water

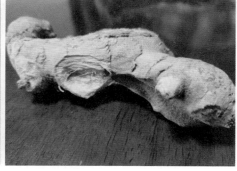

生姜

Ginger

【原料】红糖 30g，生姜 10g。

【制法】生姜去皮洗净，切丝；在锅中加入一大碗水，将切好的姜丝放入锅中开煮；待锅中水烧开后，放入红糖，用勺子搅拌均匀，大火煮 2 分钟即可。

【功效】可以发汗、解表、散寒。适用于风寒感冒初期的咳嗽、咳痰、咽痛、头痛、怕冷、身体轻度的发热等。

2. 菊花茶

【原料】干菊花 5 枚，冰糖适量。

【制法】用适量开水焖泡 25 ~ 30 分钟。

【饮法】每日 1 剂，代茶常饮。

【功效】清热、解毒、明目。

3. 银耳红枣枸杞粥

【原料】银耳 20 克，红枣 10 克，枸杞 3 克，大米适量。

【制法】银耳于温水中浸泡 30 分钟；大米淘干净，加适量的

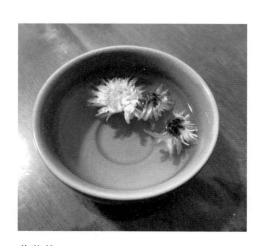

菊花茶

Juhua (Chrysanthemum Flower; Chrysanthemi Flos) Tea

水进锅中煮；15分钟左右，大米煮开，加银耳、大枣、枸杞；等到大米煮开花之后，即可食用。

【功效】补中益气、滋补肝肾。

Practical diet formulas:

1.Ginger brown sugar water

【Raw materials】Brown sugar 30g, fresh ginger 10g

【Preparation method】 Peel the fresh ginger, wash and shred; add a large bowl of water into the pot and put the shredded fresh ginger into the pot to boil. When the water in the pot boils, add brown sugar, stir evenly with a spoon, and cook over high heat for 2 minutes.

【Effect】Sweating, relieving exterior and dispersing cold. It is suitable for cough, expectoration, sore throat, headache, fear of cold, mild fever, etc.

2. Juhua (Chrysanthemum Flower; Chrysanthemi Flos) Tea

【Raw materials】5 dried chrysanthemum flowers, appropriate amount of rock sugar

【Preparation method】Soak with an appropriate amount of boiling water for 25–30 minutes.

【Drinking method】1 dose per day. Drink it often to substitute tea.

【Effects】Clearing heat, detoxifying and brightening eyes.

3. Soup of Tremella, medlar and Chinese dates

【Raw materials】Tremella 20g, Chinese dates 10g, matrimony vine 3g, and appropriate amount of rice

【Preparation method】Soak Tremella in warm water for 30 minutes; clean the rice, add an appropriate amount of water into the pot and cook for about 15 minutes. When the rice is boiled, add tremella, Chinese dates and medlar; after the rice is boiled and blossomed, it can be eaten.

【Effect】Replenish qi and nourish liver and kidney.

Chinese dietotherapy not only has a long history in China, but also has an impact on foreign countries. With the continuous improvement of people's living standards and the continuous increase of sub-health population, the emergence and development of integrated traditional Chinese and Western medicine diet is the necessity of social demand and historical development. In recent years, integrated traditional Chinese and Western medicine diet has gradually moved towards integration, accuracy, prevention priority, socialization, internationalization and economic benefit optimization, and has been paid more and more attention by the medical community.

实践活动

1. 到河南中医药大学第三附属医院治未病中心参观。

2. 品尝养生药茶或药膳。

3. 学习制作一种养生药茶或药膳。

Practical Activities

1. Visit the Preventive Treatment of Disease Department of the Third Affiliated Hospital of Henan University of Traditional Chinese Medicine.

2. Taste medicinal tea or diet.

3. Learn to make a kind of medicinal tea or medicinal diet.

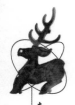

第三章　仲景文化体验与实践

中医药是中华民族的瑰宝，是打开中华文明宝库的钥匙。当前，中医药面临良好的历史发展机遇。河南是医圣张仲景的故里、仲景文化的发源地、中医药文明的发祥地，在中医药历史上具有重要地位。仲景不仅集汉代以前中国医药学之大成，还为后世中医药学创造了无限的思想动力。他所著的《伤寒杂病论》，开创了中医辨证论治的先河，奠定了中医临床治疗学的基础，历经两千余年临床实践，一直被公认为中国医学方书之鼻祖，被奉为医学经典。其理、法、方、药一直指导着中医的临床实践，历代研习者不计其数，至今依然是"道经千载更光辉"，成为祖国医学宝库中的明珠。

博大精深的张仲景医药文化，以"万世医宗"张仲景为核心，以科学严谨的治学精神、勇于创新的崇高思想、救死扶伤的优良医德为内核，千百年来，为人民群众的生命健康做出了不朽贡献，在全国乃至全世界都占有十分重要的地位。弘扬仲景文化，光大医圣精神，传播医圣文化，擦亮仲景品牌，服务全人类健康，应该是每一位中医药人的责任。

Chapter Ⅲ Experience and Practice of Zhongjing Culture

Traditional Chinese medicine is the treasure of the Chinese nation and the key to the treasure-house of Chinese civilization. At present, traditional Chinese medicine is facing a time of great historical development opportunities. Henan, the hometown of medical saint Zhang Zhongjing, the birthplace of Zhongjing culture, and the cradle of traditional Chinese medicine civilization, holds an important position in the history of traditional Chinese medicine. Zhongjing not only gathered the achievements of Chinese medicine before the Han Dynasty, but also created infinite ideological power for later generations of Chinese medicine. His *Shanghan Zabing Lun* (Treatise on Cold Damage and Miscellaneous Diseases) pioneered TCM syndrome differentiation and treatment, and laid the foundation for TCM clinical therapeutics. After over 2,000 years of clinical practice, this classic has always been regarded as the first work of Chinese medical prescriptions and a medical classic as well. have always guided the clinical practice of traditional Chinese medicine. and it is still "the classics of Taoism are more brilliant for thousands of years", becoming the pearl in the treasure house of the motherland's medicine. Its principles, methods, formula, and medicines have constantly guided the clinical

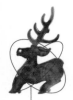

practice of traditional Chinese medicine. There are countless practitioners in the past dynasties studying and researching this classic, and until now it still has a splendid inheritance and development, becoming a pearl in the treasure-house of Chinese medicine.

The broad and profound Zhang Zhongjing's medical culture, represented by Zhang Zhongjing, takes the scientific and rigorous academic spirit, the noble thoughts of innovation, and the excellent medical ethics of saving lives and healing the wounded as its core principles. For thousands of years, it has made immortal contributions to the lives and health of the people. It occupies a very important position in the country and even the world. It should be the responsibility of every Chinese medicine practitioner to carry forward the Zhongjing culture and the spirit of the Medical Saint, spread the medical saint culture, polish the Zhongjing brand, and serve the health of all human beings.

第一节　认识医圣张仲景

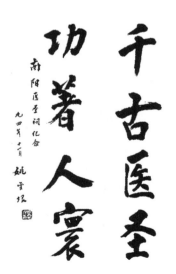

张仲景（约 150—219），名机，河南南阳人，东汉时期伟大的医学家。其所作《伤寒杂病论》对后世医学发展的影响极大，故张仲景被中外医学界尊为"医中之圣"。

张仲景自幼天资聪明，勤奋好学，酷爱读书，尤其喜爱医学著作。年仅 10 岁时的他，便师从同郡名医张伯祖，学习医术，钻研医理，得到了张伯祖毕生积累的丰富行医经验。因此，青年时期的他便医术超群、造福乡里百姓，并且仲景为人诚恳而谦虚，不论患者贫穷富贵，均有求必应，故而被举为南阳郡的孝廉，并出任长沙太守。

在长沙任内，张仲景并没有因为每日繁杂的地方政务而忽视了他对中医的热爱和钻研。一有机会，他便深入民间百姓中，观察百姓的真实状况，留心各种疾病，同时注意搜集民间流传的方剂。在闲暇时间，他会召见地方上有名的医生，与他们一同商讨医理，诚恳求教，从而得以融汇各家所长，不断丰富自己的医学知识。

公元 195 年（建安元年）以后，大规模的伤寒病开始在全国各地蔓延流行。在不到 10 年时间里，张仲景 200 多人的家族里，有 90 多人因感染伤寒而去世。"感往昔之沦丧，伤横夭之莫救"。他深知当时的医生大多数"不肯探求医经，推演新知各承家传，始终守旧"。于是，张仲景决心埋头著作，以惠及家人邻里。他认真总结前人的医学理论，根据自己丰富的临床实践并参考一生收集的大量民间方剂，经过十几年的

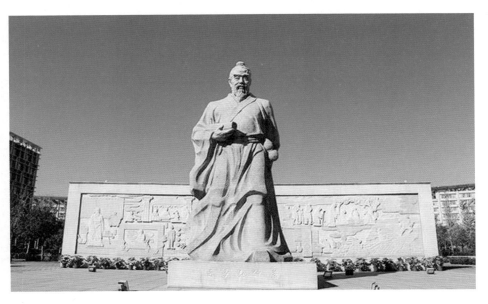

张仲景像
Zhang Zhongjing Statue

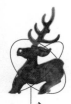

努力，终于撰写了融理、法、方、药为一体的《伤寒杂病论》。其后，该著作被分为《伤寒论》和《金匮要略》，与《黄帝内经》《神农本草经》并称为中医学的四大经典，是中国医学史上影响最大的著作之一。

Section Ⅰ   Introduction of Zhang Zhongjing

Zhang Zhongjing (about 150-219 AD) , also named Zhang Ji, was born in Nanyang, Henan Province. He was a great TCM physician in the Eastern Han Dynasty. His book *Shanghan Zabing Lun* (*Treatise on Cold Damage and Miscellaneous Diseases*) has a great influence on the development of later Chinese medicine, so Zhang Zhongjing is respected as "the Saint of Chinese Medicine".

Zhang Zhongjing was gifted and intelligent since childhood, diligent and eager to learn, and loved to read, especially medical works. When he was only 10 years old, he started to learn from Zhang Bozu, a famous doctor in the same county. He studied medical theory and skills from Zhang Bozu and gained rich medical experience. Therefore, in his youth, he already had excellent medical skills and benefited the local people. In addition, he was sincere and humble, and responded to every request no matter how poor or lowly the person was. Thus, he was promoted to be the representative of filial piety of Nanyang County and served as the prefect of Changsha.

During his tenure in Changsha, Zhang Zhongjing did not neglect his interest and research in Chinese medicine because of his daily complicated local government affairs. Whenever he had a chance, he would go deep into the people, observe the people's conditions, pay attention to various diseases, and collect folk prescriptions. In his spare time, he would summon local famous doctors to discuss medical principles and sincerely ask for advice, so as to integrate the experience of various schools and constantly enrich his medical knowledge.

After 195 AD, a large-scale epidemic began to spread throughout the country. In less than ten years, in Zhang Zhongjing's 200-people family, more than 90 of them died of the epidemic. He was well aware that most of the doctors at that time "would not seek the medical classics and deduce new knowledge, but only inherited from their own families and remained conservative all the time". Therefore, Zhang Zhongjing was determined to write a book to help his family and neighbors. He seriously summarized the previous medical theories, combined with his clinical practice, and referred to a large number of folk prescriptions collected in his life. After more than ten years of hard work, he finally wrote *Shanghan Zabing Lun* (*Treatise on Cold Damage and Miscellaneous Diseases*) which integrates treatment principles, methods, formulas, and herbal medicines. This book was divided into *Shanghan Lun* (*Treatise on Cold Damage Diseases*) and *Jingui Yaolue* (*Synopsis of the Golden Chamber*) later on. These two books together with *Huangdi Neijing* (*Huangdi's Internal Classic*) and *Shennong Bencao Jing* (*Shennong's Classic of Materia Medica*) are known as the four classics of Chinese medicine, and are the most influential works in the history of Chinese medicine.

实践活动

1. 利用图书馆等学术资源搜索张仲景及《伤寒杂病论》的相关文献，了解张仲景的杰出贡献。

2. 实地瞻仰河南中医药大学仲景广场张仲景雕像，游览河南中医药大学博物馆仲景馆。

课后作业

1. 对医圣张仲景的认识和看法，可以小组讨论。

2. 以医圣张仲景为例，谈谈中医大师的成才途径。

Practical activities

1. Search Zhang Zhongjing and related literature of *Shanghan Zabing Lun* (*Treatise on Cold Damage and Miscellaneous Diseases*) by using academic resources such as libraries to understand Zhang Zhongjing's outstanding contribution.

2. Visit the classroom of *Shanghan Zabing Lun* (*Treatise on Cold Damage and Miscellaneous Diseases*) for TCM students to understand its academic status.

Homework

1. The understanding of Zhang Zhongjing can be discussed in groups.

2. Take Zhang Zhongjing as an example to talk about the way to become a master of Traditional Chinese Medicine.

第二节　医圣仲景故事

一、吃饺子忆仲景

饺子祖始张磊

"好吃不过饺子"，饺子是中国北方传统的节日美食。饺子原名"娇耳"，民间有"十月一，冬至到，家家户户吃水饺"等耳熟能详的谚语。而这个饮食习俗的背后却隐藏着一段感人的故事，并且这个故事的主人公便是医圣张仲景。

建安初年，张仲景在告老还乡的途中，正赶上那年冬天的一场大雪，天气极其寒冷。经过白河的时候，许多穷苦的百姓面黄肌瘦，沿河乞讨，衣不蔽体，他们边走边瑟瑟发抖，有的甚至连耳朵都冻烂了。张仲景医者仁心，看到这一幕心里十分难受。

回到家后，由于张仲景远近闻名的高超医术和高尚医德，很多人上门求医。张仲景对待他们总是有求必应，悉心诊疗，虽然每天都很忙碌，但是他总是会想起那日在河边看到的场景，心里也一直牵挂着那些冻烂耳朵的穷苦百姓。

经过多次试验，张仲景发明出了一个可以御寒的食疗方。他仿照在长沙治疗瘟疫时使用大锅施药的办法，安排弟子在南阳东关的一块空地

上搭起医棚，架起大锅，向穷人免费施药治伤，开张的那天正好是冬至。他用羊肉、辣椒和一些祛寒药材在大锅里熬煮，炖熟后切成碎块，再用面把碎块包成面团，然后放入锅里煮。因为面团包完后看起来像一只耳朵，于是张仲景称其为"娇耳"，称该方为"祛寒娇耳汤"。

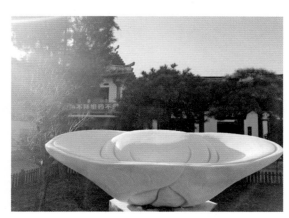

在场的穷苦百姓每人一碗热汤，两个"娇耳"，食用不久便浑身发热，血液通畅，两耳变暖。张仲景心系百姓，天天施药，一直持续到大年三十，乡亲们的耳朵也都被他治好了。因此大年初一，人们

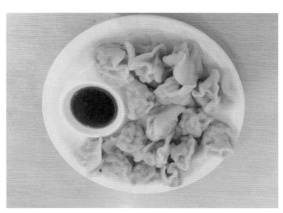

饺子
Dumpling

在庆祝新年的同时，也庆祝耳朵康复，就仿照"娇耳"的样子做过年的食物，当时为了区别"娇耳汤"的药方，就改称为"饺耳"。因叫着别嘴，后来人们就称它为"饺子"了。自此便有了冬至和大年初一吃饺子的习俗，以纪念张仲景开棚施药和治愈病人的日子。

"祛寒娇耳汤"的故事一直在民间流传，南阳当地的老人至今仍然在冬至的时候告诫那些不喜欢吃饺子的小孩儿："冬至不端饺子碗，冻掉耳朵没人管。"质朴的语言饱含着浓浓的感恩情怀。

Section II Zhongjing's Story

I. Zhang Zhongjing and Dumplings

"There's nothing more delicious than dumplings." Dumpling is a traditional festival food in northern China. The original name of dumpling was "Jiao-er", which means delicate ears. There are well-known proverbs among the people, such as "October 1st, the Winter Solstice, every family eats dumplings". There is a touching story behind this dietary custom, and the protagonist is the "Saint of Chinese Medicine" Zhang Zhongjing.

Zhang Zhongjing once served as the prefect of Changsha, and later resigned and returned to his hometown to treat his neighbors. On his way home, he caught up with a heavy snowfall that winter, and it was weather was extremely cold. When passing through the Baihe River, many poor people were pale and skinny, begging along the river, and their clothes were scanty. They shivered as they walked, and some even had their ears frozen. Doctor Zhang Zhongjing was benevolent and felt very sad when he saw this scene.

After returning home, many people came to Zhongjing's house and sought medical treatment due to his famous superb medical skills and noble medical ethics. Zhang Zhongjing always responded to their requests and treated them carefully. Although he was very busy every day, he always remembered the scene he saw by the river that day and worried about the poor people with frozen ears.

After many experiments, Zhang Zhongjing invented a diet that can keep out the cold. He imitated the method of using a big pot to deliver herbal medicine when treating the plague in Changsha, and arranged his disciples to set up a medical shed and a big pot in an open space of Nanyang, Dongguan, to give free herbal medicine to the poor. The opening day was the Winter Solstice. He boiled mutton, pepper and some cold-dispelling herbs in a big pot. After stewing, he cut the mutton into pieces, wrapped it in dough and put it into the pot. Because the dough looked like an ear after wrapping, Zhang Zhongjing called it "Jiao-er", which means delicate ear in Chinese, and called the recipe "Jiao-er Soup to keep out the cold".

The poor people on the scene each had a bowl of hot soup and two "delicate ears". Soon after eating, they were hot all over. Their blood was unobstructed, and their ears got warm. Zhang Zhongjing was so concerned about the people and applied the soup every day until the New Year's Eve, and the villagers' ears were cured by him. Therefore, on the first day of the Lunar New Year, people celebrated the new year as well as the recovery of frozen ears. They made new year's food in the same way as "Jiao-er". At that time, in order to distinguish the prescription of "Jiao-er Soup", the food was renamed "Jiao-er", with the same sound but different character. Later people called it "Jiaozi" in Chinese because it's easier to speak. Since then, there has been the custom of eating dumplings (Jiaozi) on the Winter Solstice and the first day of the Lunar New Year to commemorate the day when Zhang Zhongjing cooked the decoction and cured the patients.

The story of "Jiao-er Soup" has been popular among the people. The local elders in Nanyang still warn children who don't like dumplings during the Winter Solstice: "If you don't bring dumpling bowls during the Winter Solstice, no one will care if you freeze your ears." It's a simple proverb, but full of a strong sense of gratitude to Zhang Zhongjing.

实践活动

1. 参加一次包饺子实践活动，体验饺子的形状和文化内涵。

2. 实地考察南阳当地的饺子馆，了解当地的饺子习俗。

课后作业

1. 对饺子的印象或看法，可以书面形式发表感悟。

2. 以小组讨论方式谈谈中医与饺子的联系。

Practical activities

1. Participate in a dumpling making practice to experience the cultural connotation of dumplings.

2. Visit the local dumpling restaurant in Nanyang to understand the local dumpling customs.

Homework

1. The impression or opinion of dumplings can be expressed in written form.

2. Talk about the relationship between Traditional Chinese Medicine and dumplings through group discussion.

二、仲景驳斥巫术

旧社会迷信盛行，有些人生了病不是去找医生，而是请男巫或女巫用巫术治病，结果既花去不少钱，又因得不到有效治疗而被病魔夺去生命。张仲景对这些巫医非常痛恨，每次遇到他们装神弄鬼、误人性命，就出面干预，并用疗效来驳斥巫术迷信，奉劝人们相信医术。有一次，他遇见一个妇女，总是疑神疑鬼，一会哭一会笑。病人家属听信巫婆的谎言，以为是"鬼怪缠身"，要请巫婆为她"驱邪"。张仲景碰巧遇到，就阻止了巫婆的做法，用中医治疗该病人。张仲景观察了病人的气色和病态，又询问了病人的有关情况，然后对病人家属说："她根本不是什么鬼怪缠身，而是因受到较大刺激造成的，属于中医上所说的'热血入室'。她的病完全可以治好。真正的鬼怪是那些可恶的巫婆，千万不能让她们缠住病人，否则病人会有性命危险。"在征得病人家属同意后，他为病人针刺了期门，并给病人开了几付中药。几天后，那妇女的病就慢慢好起来，疑鬼疑神的症状也消失了。从此，一些人生了病，便不再相信巫医的鬼话，而是找张仲景治病。

课后作业：

1. 了解世界医学史中巫医的兴起与消亡。
2. 查阅《伤寒论》中"热入血室"的诊断与治疗。

II. Zhongjing refuted the witchcraft

Superstition prevailed in the old society, and some people who fell ill did not go to see the doctor, but asked witch doctors to use witchcraft to cure diseases. As a result, they spent a lot of money but were killed by the disease because they could not get effective treatment. Zhang Zhongjing hated these witch doctors a lot, and each time he encountered them pretending to be ghosts and mistaking people's lives, he intervened, and used curative effects to refute the superstition of witchcraft and persuade people to believe in medical skills. Once, he met a woman who was always suspicious and would cry and laugh. The patient's family believed the witch's lies, thought it was "haunted by ghosts", and asked the witch to "exorcise evil" for her. By chance, Zhang Zhongjing happened to be there, and he stopped the witch doctor and used

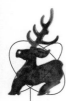
traditional Chinese medicine to treat the patient. Zhang Zhongjing observed the patient's appearance and condition, asked about the patient's relevant information, and then said to the patient's family: "She is not haunted by ghosts at all, but experienced great emotional triggers. Her condition belongs to what Chinese medicine calls 'hot blood entering the body *Xue Shi*'. Her illness could be cured. The real ghosts are the hateful witches, and they must not be allowed to entangle the patient, otherwise the patient's life will be in danger." After obtaining the consent of the patient's family, he did acupuncture on the patient at Qimen point and prescribed several Chinese medicines to the patient. After a few days, the woman's condition slowly improved, and the symptoms of suspiciousness disappeared. Since then, some people who have been sick no longer believe the witch doctor's lies, but seek Zhang Zhongjing to treat their disease.

三、仲景巧医心病

张仲景在医学上出了名后，仍旧为人谦虚，一点也不摆名医的架子；同时，他还虚心地为同行医病，不失时机地向别的郎中学习。

从前的一些郎中们，只把医术与秘方传给自己的子孙，一般都不外传。那时南阳有个名医叫沈槐，已经 70 多岁了，还没有子女。他整天惆怅后继无人，饭吃不下，觉睡不着，慢慢忧虑成病了。

当地的郎中们，来给沈槐看病，都没有很好的医治方法。老先生的病谁也看不好，越来越重了。张仲景知道后，就专门来到沈槐家里为他医治。

张仲景察看了病情，确诊这是忧虑成疾，马上开了一个药方，用五谷杂粮面各一斤，团成圆球形，外边涂上朱砂，叫病人一顿食完。

沈槐知道后，心里感觉十分好笑。他命家人把那五谷杂粮面做成药丸，挂在屋檐下，逢人就指着这药丸把张仲景奚落一番。

亲戚来看他时，他笑着说："看！这是张仲景给我开的药方。谁见过五谷杂粮能医病？笑话！笑话！"

朋友来看他时，他笑着说："看！这是张仲景给我开的药方，谁一顿能吃五斤面，真滑稽！滑稽！"

同行的郎中来看他时，他笑着说："看！这是张仲景给我开的药方。我看几十年病，听就没听说过，真是好笑。"

他一心只想这件事可笑，忧心多虑的事全抛脑后了，不知不觉地病就好了。

这时，张仲景来拜访他，说："恭喜先生的病好了！学生斗胆在鲁班门前弄斧了。"沈槐一听恍然大悟，又佩服，又惭愧。张仲景接着又说："先生，我们做郎中的，就是为了给百姓造福，祛病延年，先生无子女，我们这些年轻人不都是你的子女吗？何愁后继无人？"沈槐听了，觉得很有道理，内心十分感动。

从此，就把自己的医术全部传授给了张仲景和其他年轻的郎中。

Ⅲ. Zhang Zhongjing treated mental illness skillfully

After Zhang Zhongjing became famous in medicine, he was still modest and did not pretend to be a famous doctor at all. At the same time, he also humbly treated his peers and grasped opportunity to learn from other physicians trained in herbal medicine .

In the past, some physicians only passed on medical skills and secret recipes to their descendants, and generally did not spread to strangers. At that time, there was a famous doctor named Shen Huai in Nanyang who was in his seventies and had no offspring. He was sad all day long since he worried about having no successor. He couldn't eat, sleep and became worried and fell ill finally.

The local physicians came to see Shen Huai, but there was no good way to treat Shen Huai. No one can treat the old man's illness well, which made

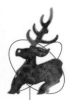

the illness more and more serious. After Zhang Zhongjing knew about it, he specially came to Shen Huai's house to treat him.

Zhang Zhongjing inspected the condition and confirmed that it was caused by worry. He immediately prescribed a prescription. He used one catty of grain noodles, which was reunited into a ball, coated with bead sand outside, and asked the patient to eat it with a meal .

After Shen Huai knew about it, he felt very ridiculous . He ordered his family to hang the pill made of grain noodles under the eaves, and every time when people came he would point to this pill and taunted Zhang Zhongjing.

When relatives came to see him, he smiled and said, "Look! This is the prescription prescribed by Zhang Zhongjing. Who has ever seen that grains and miscellaneous grains can cure diseases? Joke! Joke!"

When his friends came to see him, he smiled and said, "Look! This is the prescription prescribed by Zhang Zhongjing for me. It's so laughable that who can eat five catties of noodles at a meal! Funny! Funny!"

When colleagues came to see him, he smiled and said, "Look! This is the prescription prescribed by Zhang Zhongjing. I have been treating people for decades, but I have never heard of it. It's really funny." It's so ridiculous for him to only think about this and forgot all his worries that the ill recovered unconsciously. He always thought about this prescription and...

At this time, Zhang Zhongjing came to visit him and said, "Congratulations, teacher, for getting well! I dared to teach fish to swim." As soon as Shen Huai heard this, he suddenly realized what had happened,admired Zhang Zhongjing, and felt ashamed. Zhang Zhongjing went on to say, "Teacher, we as doctors should benefit the people and prolong the sicknesses. Although you have no children, aren't we your children? Why did you worry that you have no successors?" When Shen Huai heard this, he felt very reasonable and was very moved.

Since then, he taught all medical skills to Zhang Zhongjing and other young physicians.

课后作业

1. 查阅文献谈谈中医对精神情志病的常用方法。

2. 谈谈你对精神情志疗法的理解。

Homework

1. Consult literature and talk about the common methods of treating mental illness in traditional Chinese medicine.

2. Talk about your understanding of psychopathic therapy.

四、仲景求学叔父

仲景从小天资聪明，勤奋好学。张仲景的同族叔叔张伯祖是当时南阳一带的名医，经常四处给人治病。

有一天，邻村一名农民得了伤寒病，来请张伯祖去诊治。正巧张仲景在叔父家里，于是张伯祖便带着仲景一起去给病人诊治。经过用药，患者很快痊愈了。张仲景亲眼看到叔父这高超的医术，心里赞叹不已。他十分羡慕地问："叔父的医道这么高明，是怎么学来的？"张伯祖听了，笑笑说："我行医这么多年，也没有什么经验可说，但是悟出一个道理，那就是：要想成为一个医生，必须勤求古训，博采众方。"张仲景恍然大悟，于是拜张伯祖为师下功夫钻研医药，精究方术，决心做一个能"上以疗君亲之疾，下以救贫贱之厄，中以保身长全"的好医生。

从此以后，张仲景每天除了在家钻研医书之外，一有机会，就跟着张伯祖外出治病，通过实践来验证从书本上学到的医学理论，加深对医药理论的理解，丰富自己的临床经验。虚心诚恳地请张伯祖传授医术。这样，不知不觉三年过去了，张伯祖看张仲景这样勤奋好学，心里有说

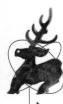

不出的高兴，便把自己的所有本事都传授给他。

十几岁的张仲景拜张伯祖为师，勤奋钻研医术决心为民除疾的事，很快在南阳郡传开了。一天，仲景去拜访同郡一位当时在朝中名人何颙，何颙和他交谈以后，发现他的志向十分坚定，非常饮佩地对张仲景说："你这样热爱医学，又这样聪明而勤奋，将来长大后不论做官还是写诗词文章都不一定能有多大成就。但是，你一定能成为一个有名的好医生。"仲景听了笑着说："进则救世，退则救民，不能为良相，亦当为良医。"

课后作业

1. 了解中医对伤寒病的看法。

2. 谈谈对"不能为良相，亦当为良医"的认识。

IV. Zhongjing was apprenticed to his uncle for traditional Chinese medicine

Zhongjing grew up with natural intelligence and was diligent in learning. As a famous doctor in Nanyang, Zhang Zhongjing's uncle Zhang Bozu often healed the sick everywhere at that time.

One day, a farmer in a neighboring village got typhoid fever and asked Zhang Bozu to treat him. It happened that Zhang Zhongjing was at his uncle's house, so Zhang Bozu took Zhongjing with him to treat the patient. After medication, the patient was quickly cured. Seeing his uncle's superb medical skills with his own eyes, Zhang Zhongjing was overwhelmed with admiration. He asked with great envy, "How did you learn to be so skilled in medicine, uncle?" Zhang Bozu smiled and said, "I have been practicing medicine for so many years, and I have no experience to speak of, but I have learned one thing: To become a doctor, one must diligently seek ancient teachings and learn from all sides." Zhang Zhongjing suddenly understood realized, so he worshipped/

Zhang Bozu as his teacher and made great effort to study medicine and prescriptions, determined to be a good doctor who could "treat the illnesses of the ruler's relatives, save help the poor and lowly people's difficulties, and keep his body intact".

From then on, in addition to studying medical books at home every day, Zhang Zhongjing would follow Zhang Bozu out to treat patients whenever he had the chance, to verify the medical theories he learned from books through practice, to deepen his understanding of medical theories and to enrich his clinical experience. He humbly and sincerely asked Zhang Bozu to teach him the art of medicine. In this way, unknowingly, three years passed. Seeing how diligent Zhang Zhongjing was in learning, Zhang Bozu was so happy that he taught him all his skills.

As a teenager, Zhang Zhongjing worshipped Zhang Bozu as his teacher, diligently studied medical skills and was determined to eliminate diseases for the people, which soon spread in Nanyang County. One day, Zhongjing went to visit a famous person in the same county, He Yong, who was in the court at that time. After talking with him, He Yong found his ambition very strong and said to Zhang Zhongjing with great admiration: "You are so passionate about medicine and so smart and diligent. You may not be able to achieve much when you grow up, no matter you are a government official or write poems and articles. However, you will definitely become a famous and good doctor." Zhongjing smiled and said, "If I enter the world, I will save the world; if I retreat, I will save the people; if I can't be a good minister, I will be a good doctor."

Homework

1. Learn Understand the views of Chinese medicine on typhoid fever.

2. Talk about your understanding of "if you are not a good doctor, you should be a good doctor".

五、"坐堂医"张仲景

张仲景在任长沙太守期间，正值疫病流行，许多贫苦百姓慕名前来求医。他对前来求医者总是热情接待，细心诊治，从不拒绝。开始他是在处理完公务之后，在后堂或自己家中给人治病；后来，前来治病者越来越多，使他应接不暇，于是他干脆把诊所搬到了长沙大堂，公开坐堂应诊，首创了名医坐大堂的先例，他的这一举动被传为千古佳话。

后来，人民为了怀念张仲景，便把坐在药店内治病的医生通称为"坐堂医"。这些医生也把自己开设的药店取名为"××堂药店"，这就是中医药店称"堂"的来历。

Ⅴ. Zhang Zhongjing, the "Sitting Doctor"

When Zhang Zhongjing was the governor of Changsha, there was an epidemic and many poor people came to him for medical treatment. In contrast to the official style of the feudal court officials, he always received those who came to him warmly and treated them carefully, and never refused. At first, he treated people in the back room or in his own home after dealing with his official duties. Later, as more and more people came to treat the disease, he was overwhelmed, so he simply moved his clinic to the lobby of Changsha and sat in the lobby openly, setting a precedent for famous doctors to sit in the lobby. His move was passed down as a good story through the ages.

Later, in order to commemorate Zhang Zhongjing, people called the doctors who sat in the pharmacies to treat patients as "sitting doctors". These doctors also named their own pharmacies "××Tang Pharmacy", which is the origin of the name "Tang" for Chinese medicine stores.

实践活动

1. 实地参观张仲景大药房。

2. 体验坐堂中医诊疗服务。

课后作业

1. 对张仲景大药房的印象或看法，可以小组讨论。

2. 通过自媒体宣传张仲景大药房坐堂场景。

Practical activities

1. Field trip to Zhang Zhongjing Pharmacy.

2. Experience the service of sitting in a Chinese medicine shop.

Homework

1. Impressions or opinions of Zhang Zhongjing Pharmacy, which can be discussed in groups./You can say your views or opinions about Zhongjing Pharmacy through group discussion.

2. Promote Zhang Zhongjing Pharmacy through self media.

第三节　仲景两大医学成就

一、仲景首创六经

辨证论治是中医学的基本原则，具有显明的特色与优势，而张仲景是辨证论治的首创者。中国最早的古典医籍《内经》已经有了辨证论治思想，但还未形成完整的理论体系。因为辨证论治包括"辨证"与"论治"两大部分，必须体现理、法、方、药的一致性、连贯性、完整性，而《内经》显然还未达到，特别是论治部分更为欠缺，但在张仲景的《伤寒杂病论》中已处处得到体现。从近年来在内蒙居延、甘肃武威和长沙马王堆出土的汉代医学简牍来看，这些稍早于张仲景的文物也未达到这一高度。所以说张仲景才能称得上是辨证论治的首创者。具体表现在以下两方面：

第一，《伤寒论》是我国第一部系统阐述外感病辨证论治的专书。它在《素问·热论》六经分证的基础上，对外感病的发生、发展、变化和防治进行了深入细致的探讨，创造性地提出了"六经辨证"的理论，不仅对外感病，而且对临床各科均具有临床指导作用。

第二，八纲辨证是辨证论治的基本方法和主要内容之一，八纲辨证的创始人是张仲景。在《伤寒杂病论》中虽然找不到"八纲"这一具体的名称，但它已经体现了八纲的具体内容和精神实质。在《伤寒论》各篇中，六经病证与八纲的关系是十分密切的，全书所论所辨均不出阴阳、表里、寒热、虚实八纲的圈子。《伤寒论》不但处处贯串着八纲的内容，而且辨证与论治运用得灵活自如，相互交错，相互渗透，形成了一个完整的辨证论治的理论体系。

此外，从《伤寒杂病论》中可以看到脏腑辨证的萌芽。《金匮要略》的第一篇就是以"脏腑经络先后病脉证第一"命名的。其他各篇有不少病证也是以脏腑学说作为辨证论治的说理工具。从《伤寒论》六经辨证的实际内容来看，太阳病（腑证）与膀胱有关，阳明病主要就是指胃肠的病变，少阳病与胆密切相关，太阴病即脾的虚寒证，少阴病指心肾的病变，厥阴病与心包、肝有某种联系。这些内容对后世脏腑辨证理论的形成和发展肯定有启示作用。

Section III Zhongjing's two major medical achievements

ⅼ. Zhongjing created the theory of six meridians

Zhang Zhongjing pioneered the treatment based on syndrome differentiation with its obvious characteristics and strengths, which is the basic principle of Chinese medicine. *Nei Jing*, the earliest medical book in China, already has the thought of syndrome differentiation and treatment, but it has not yet formed a complete theoretical system.

Nei Jing has not reached the treatment part. especially the treatment part is even more lacking. But it has been reflected everywhere in *Shanghan Zabing Lun* (*Treatise on Cold Damage and Miscellaneous Diseases*). Judging from the medical slips of the Han Dynasty unearthed in Juyan in Inner Mongolia, Wuwei in Gansu and Mawangdui in Changsha in recent years, these cultural relics earlier than Zhang Zhongjing have not reached this level. Therefore, Zhang Zhongjing can be regarded as the pioneer of syndrome differentiation and treatment. It is embodied in the following two aspects.

Firstly, *Shanghan Zabing Lun* (*Treatise on Cold Damage and Miscellaneous Diseases*) is the first book in China that systematically expounds the syndrome differentiation and treatment of exogenous diseases. On the basis of the six-meridian and syndrome differentiation in *Su Wen* (*Plain Questions*), it conducts in-depth and meticulous discussions on the occurrence, development, change and prevention of externally susceptible diseases, and creatively puts forward the theory of six-meridian syndrome differentiation. Additionally, it has a clinical guiding role for not only external infection, but also for all clinical departments.

Secondly, the eight-principle syndrome differentiation is one of the basic methods and main contents of syndrome differentiation and treatment, whose founder is Zhang Zhongjing. Although the specific name of Eight-Principle cannot be found in *Shanghan Zabing Lun* (*Treatise on Cold Damage and Miscellaneous Diseases*), it has already reflected the specific content and spiritual essence of the Eight Principles. In each chapter of *Shanghan Lun* (*Treatise on Cold Damage Diseases*), the relationship between the six-meridian and the eight-principle is very close, and the whole book discusses and distinguishes within the area of *yin* and *yang*, outer and inner, cold and heat, deficiency and excess. *Shanghan Lun* (*Treatise on Cold Damage Diseases*) not only runs through the contents of the Eight-Principle, but also its application of syndrome differentiation and treatment is flexible, intertwined and penetrated, forming a complete theoretical system of syndrome differentiation and treatment.

In addition, we can see the germination of Zang-fu（脏腑）syndrome differentiation in *Shanghan Zabing Lun* (*Treatise on Cold Damage and Miscellaneous Diseases*). The first chapter of *Jingui Yaolue* (*Synopsis of the Golden Chamber*) is termed "脏腑经络先后病脉证第一". In other chapters, many diseases and syndromes are also based on the theory of Zang-fu（脏腑学说）as a theoretical tool for syndrome differentiation and treatment. Judging from the content of the six-meridian syndrome differentiation in *Shanghan Lun* (*Treatise on Cold Damage Taiyang Disease*), Taiyang Disease (Fu syndrome) is related to the bladder, Yangming Disease mainly refers to the lesions of the gastrointestinal tract, Shaoyang Disease is closely related to the gallbladder, and Taiyin Disease is the deficiency of the spleen, Shaoyin Disease refers to the issues of the heart and kidney, and Jueyin Disease has some connection with the pericardium and liver. These contents will definitely have enlightenment for the formation and development of the theory of Zang-fu differentiation for later generations.

课后作业

1. 了解中医几种常见的辨证方法。

2. 谈谈对六经辨证的认识。

Homework

1. Understand several common syndrome differentiation methods in TCM;

2.Talk about the understanding of the six classics dialectics.

二、方剂鼻祖仲景

《伤寒论》载方 113 方，《金匮要略》载方 205 方。书中不少有名方剂，千百年来一直被历代医家沿用于治疗临床各科疾病，而且具有较高的疗效。故后世医家把《伤寒杂病论》赞誉为"方书之祖"，对后世方剂学的发展影响甚大。

在药剂方面，《伤寒论》与《金匮要略》二书中的剂型就有十余种，不但在数量上比《内经》大有增加（《内经》只有五六种剂型），而且在制剂方面也有了很多充实与发展。

张仲景对汤剂的煎煮方法、服药方法等均很重视，记载颇详。煎煮方法有先煎、后下、分煎、去渣再煎、沸水渍泡等。煎药的用水也各有所异，如清水、甘澜水、麻沸汤、清浆水、潦水、泉水、井花水、醋水合煎、水酒合煎等。

《伤寒论》与《金匮要略》所载丸剂的制作方法有两大类，一类是直接丸法，一类是加料丸法。散剂也有二类制作方法：一是直接将药物研磨为散的，二是将药物经煅烧炮炙后再研成散的。其他如导剂、酒剂、熏剂、洗剂、膏剂、坐药、擦剂、搐鼻剂等，内容较为丰富，有许多创见，成为后世药剂发展的先声。

方剂学还包括治疗方法的内容。中医治法虽多，但一般可以"八法"概言之。虽然八法内容在《内经》中早已提出，而《伤寒杂病论》并无专章论述，但仔细研读，八法却历历在目，如麻桂之汗法、承气之下法、柴胡之和法等。说明仲景将八法具体地运用于辨证论治之中，成就是很大的。

课后作业

1. 了解《伤寒杂病论》对中医方剂学的贡献。

2. 谈谈对中医八法的认识。

II. The originator of the prescription: Zhongjing

Shanghan Zabing Lun (*Treatise on Cold Damage and Miscellaneous Diseases*) contains 113 prescriptions, while *Jingui Yaolue* (*Synopsis of the Golden Chamber*) contains 205 prescriptions. There are many famous prescriptions in *Shanghan Zabing Lun* (*Treatise on Cold Damage and Miscellaneous Diseases*) and have been used by successive generations of doctors for the treatment of clinical diseases for thousands of years, and have a high efficacy. Because of this, *Shanghan Zabing Lun* (*Treatise on Cold Damage and Miscellaneous Diseases*) was praised by later generations of medical scientists as the "originator of the prescription", and have a great influence on the development of prescription science in later generations.

In terms of pharmacy, there are more than ten different forms of drug production in this two books, *Shanghan Zabing Lun* (*Treatise on Cold Damage and Miscellaneous Diseases*) and *Jingui Yaolue* (*Synopsis of the Golden Chamber*), which not only greatly increased in quantity over the *Su Wen* (*Plain Questions*) of *Huangdi Neijing* (*Huangdi's Internal Classic*) , but also enriched and developed a lot in the production of medicinal agents.

Zhang Zhongjing attached great importance to the method of making decoction and taking medicine, which was quite detailed in *Shanghan Zabing Lun* (*Treatise on Cold Damage and Miscellaneous Diseases*). The methods of decoction vary depending on theherb itself or the purpose of the formula, including being decocted first, being decocted later, being decocted separately, being decocted after removing the residues and being soaked in the boiled water, etc. The water used for decoction also varies, such as clear water, water with bubbles rolling on the surface, simmering water, clear fermented sour water, accumulated water after the rain, spring water, water in the early morning, vinegar combined with water, water combined with wine, etc.

There are two major types of pill production methods seen in *Shanghan Lun* (*Treatise on Cold Damage Diseases*) and the "Outline of the Golden Plateau", of which one is the direct pill method, and the other is the addition pill method. And there are also two methods of powders, of which one is to directly grind the drug into a scatter, and the other is to grind the drug into a scatter after being calcined. There are also other creative pharmaceutical methods and have become the precursors of the development of later generations of pharmacies, such as alcohol extracts, ointments, plaster, etc. Prescription science also includes the content of treatment methods. Although there are many traditional Chinese medicine treatment methods, generally they can be summarized in the "Eight Methods". The "Eight Methods" has been put forward in *Su Wen* (*Plain Questions*) of *Huangdi Neijing (Huangdi's Internal Classic)*, but there is no special chapter in *Shanghan Zabing Lun* (*Treatise on Cold Damage and Miscellaneous Diseases*).

However, as long as we make a carefully study, the "Eight Methods" also can be found in *Shanghan Zabing Lun* (*Treatise on Cold Damage and Miscellaneous Diseases*) such as perspire method in Mahuang Decoction and Guizhi Decoction, purgation method in Chengqi Decoction, harmony method in Xiao Chaihu Decoction and so on, which shows that Zhang Zhongjing's concrete application of the "Eight" Laws to dialectical arguments is a great achievement.

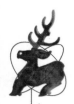

第四节　河南南阳医圣祠

　　南阳医圣祠，又名张仲景博物院，位于中国历史文化名城河南省南阳市的城东温凉河畔，它是我国东汉时期伟大的医学家、世界医史伟人、被人们尊为中华"医圣"的张仲景的墓祠纪念地。

　　医圣祠坐北朝南，占地约 11 330 平方米。它在明清时期被多次扩展，但没有确切的文献支撑其成立年份。1949 年新中国成立后，医圣祠也进行了多次修葺，并设立张仲景纪念馆，陈列展出他的生平和医学成就，为全国重点文物保护单位。

　　医圣祠大门为仿汉建筑，一对子母阙矗立在大门前，气势宏伟，阙上的彩绘朱雀傲视蓝天，翩翩欲飞。正院有山门、中殿、两庑（wǔ）；偏院有医圣井、医圣桥、素问亭、历代名医塑像等等。山门后面是张仲景陵墓，陵墓前有刻着"东汉长沙太守医圣张仲景之墓"的石碑。仲景

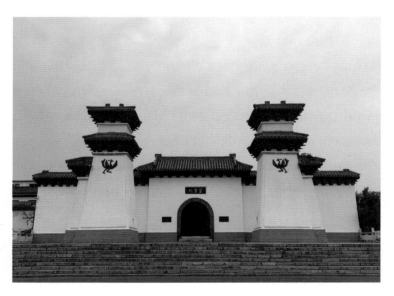

医圣祠大门
The gate of the Nanyang Medical Saint Temple

墓为汉砖砌成的正方形大理石墓基，四角镶嵌着寓意吉祥的羊头。庄严肃穆的陵墓被花墙环绕，凉亭盖顶。墓前建有拜殿，后为墓亭，各种祭祀活动均在此进行。仲景墓亭东西两侧建有行方斋、智圆斋、仁术馆、广济馆等。墓后为清代四合院式的建筑，设有医圣张仲景像以及晋唐的名医王叔和、孙思邈的塑像。西院有医圣井、荷花池、池心亭等多个游览景点。这里因亭台轩谢，风光旖旎，吸引着大批国内外游客前来观光游览。自 1988 年以来，医圣祠先后入选全国重点文物保护单位、"河南省非物质文化遗产"、"全国中医药文化教育基地"等。

医圣祠三宝

1. 东汉女体针灸陶人

"中原百件国宝文物"中的珍品，该型号高 24 厘米，宽 7 厘米，形状非常简单，但具有极高的学术价值。它比针灸专家王伟义在宋代设计的针灸铜人早了近一千年。它的艺术价值也很高，并被编入《中国美术全集》。此针灸陶人的复制品在中国历史博物馆展出。

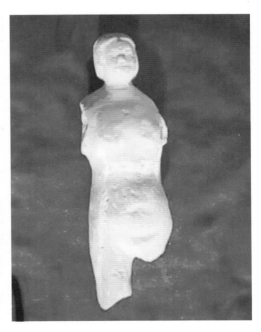

东汉女体针灸陶人

The female acupuncture pottery model of the eastern Han Dynasty

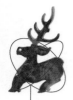

2. 东晋医圣张仲景墓碑

历经 1600 余年仍完好无损。晋碑立于公元 330 年，距医圣逝世只有 111 年。石碑上的碑文雄伟典雅，文字线条流畅，具有极高的学术、历史和艺术价值。

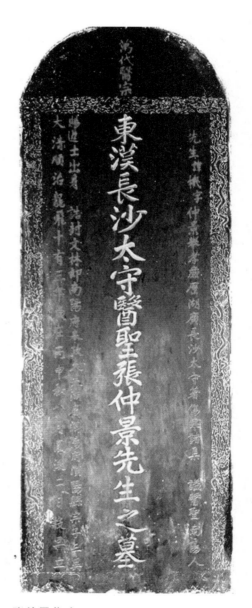

张仲景墓碑

The tombstone of Medical Saint Zhang Zhongjing

3. 白云阁藏本木刻版
《伤寒杂病论》

　　该书为张仲景第 46
代孙张绍祖所珍藏，为孤
本。1982 年陕西省中医研
究院院长米伯让根据其师
黄竹斋的遗嘱赠予南阳医
圣祠。医学家称这套木刻
版为善版、珍版、绝版。

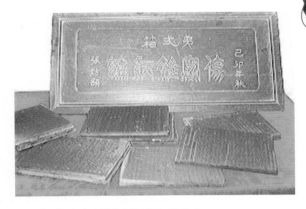

白云阁藏本木刻版《伤寒杂病论》

The woodcut edition of *Treatise on Cold Damage and Miscellaneous Diseases* in the Baiyun Pavilion Collection

Section IV　The Medical Saint Temple in Nanyang of Henan Province

The Nanyang Medical Saint Temple (Zhang Zhongjing Museum) is located by the Wenliang River in the east of Nanyang City, Henan Province. It is the memorial site of the "Saint of Chinese Medicine" Zhang Zhongjing, who was a great medical scientist in the Eastern Han Dynasty, and also a great person in the world's medical history.

The Medical Saint Temple faces south, and covers an area of about 2.8 acres. It was expanded many times in the Ming and Qing dynasties, yet there is no exact literature reference for its founding year. After liberation, the party and the state attached great importance to the protection of the medical cultural heritage and cultural relics of the motherland, and the temple was repaired many times.

At present, the gate of the Medical Saint Temple is an imitation of Han Dynasty architecture. A pair of magnificent and resplendent son-and-mother watchtowers stand in front of the gate, and the painted vermilion bird on the watchtowers looks up to the blue sky and wants to fly gracefully. The main courtyard has a mountain gate, a middle hall and two houses. In the side yard, there are Medical Holy Well, Medical Holy Bridge, Suwen Pavilion, etc. Behind the mountain gate of the main courtyard is Zhang Zhongjing's mausoleum, in front of which is a stone tablet erected by Zhang Sanyi, the Minister of Nanyang Prefecture in the 13th year of Shunzhi. On the stone tablet writes "the tomb of Zhang Zhongjing, the Medical Saint of Changsha in the Eastern Han Dynasty". The mausoleum is a square marble tomb base, built of Han bricks, with sheep's heads inlaid at the four corners, which means auspiciousness. Surrounded by flower walls and covered by a pavilion, the solemn mausoleum makes people think of ancient times with infinite admiration. There is a hall of worship in the front, and another tomb pavilion in the back, where all kinds of worship activities can be carried out. On the east and west sides of Zhongjing Tomb Pavilion are several rooms called Xingfang Zhai, Zhiyuan Zhai, Renshu Hall, Guangji Hall, etc. Behind the tomb is a Qing Dynasty courtyard-style building, where stands the statues of Zhang Zhongjing and two other famous doctors of the Jin and Tang dynasties, Wang Shuhe and Sun Simiao. There are many tourist attractions in the west yard, such as Yishengjing, lotus pool, Chixinting, etc. The pavilions are graceful and beautiful, with green trees and flowers adding more attraction. It is a fairyland in the world and attracts a large number of tourists from China and abroad. Since 1988, the Medical Saint Temple has been selected as one of the national key cultural relics protection units, "and was regarded as the Intangible Cultural Heritage of Henan Province", "National Cultural Education Base of

Traditional Chinese Medicine", and so on.

The Three Treasures of the Medical Saint Temple

The female body acupuncture pottery model of the Eastern Han Dynasty: a treasure among the "100 National Treasures of the Central Plains". This model is 24cm high and 7cm wide, very simple in shape but with extremely high academic value. It is nearly one thousand years earlier than the acupuncture bronze figurine designed by acupuncture expert Wang Weiyi in the Song Dynasty. Its artistic value is also very high, and has been included in the *Complete Works of Chinese Art*. The replica of this acupuncture pottery is on display at the Chinese History Museum.

The tombstone of Medical Saint Zhang Zhongjing: The tombstone is still intact after more than 1600 years. It was erected in 330 AD, only 111 years from the year of Zhongjing's death. The inscription on the stele is majestic and elegant, and the characters are smooth and delicate. It has high academic value, historical value and artistic value.

The woodcut edition of *Shanghan Zabing Lun* (*Treatise on Cold Damage and Miscellaneous Diseases*) in the Baiyun Pavilion Collection: It was collected by Zhang Shaozu, the 46th grandson of Zhang Zhongjing and is the unique copy. In 1982, Mi Borang, the president of Shanxi Academy of Traditional Chinese Medicine presented it to Nanyang Medical Saint Temple in accordance with the will of his teacher Huang Zhuzhai. Medical experts called the woodcut edition "a good edition", "a rare edition" and "an out-of-print edition".

实践活动

1. 实地参观南阳医圣祠，感悟仲景文化。

2. 观看或查阅医圣祠的文字或视频资料，了解医圣祠三宝。

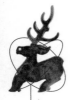

课后作业

1. 对医圣祠及仲景文化的印象或看法，可以小组讨论。

2. 向馆方申请，完成南阳医圣祠内文物的拍照或摄影。

Practical activities

1. Visit the Nanyang Medical Saint Temple and experience its culture.

2. Consult or watch the relevant literature or video materials of the Medical Saint Temple to understand its three treasures.

Homework

1. The impression or views on the Nanyang Medical Saint Temple and Zhongjing culture can be discussed in groups.

2. Take photos of cultural relics in the Nanyang Medical Saint Temple.

第五节　观览仲景文化节

仲景文化节是河南尤其南阳等地"传承仲景学术、弘扬中医文化"的重要途径，当前该文化节活动主要以"中国南阳张仲景医药科技文化节"和"河南中医药大学仲景文化节"最为著名。

中国南阳张仲景医药科技文化节前身为张仲景医药文化节，始于2002年，至2020年已成功举办了14届。南阳张仲景医药科技文化节由国家科技部、国家中医药管理局和河南省人民政府主办，旨在"传承仲景学术、弘扬中医国粹"，其活动主要包括"中医药科技创新与产业化发展战略论坛""中医药科技创新与产业化发展成果展览""中医药文化建设研讨""张仲景经方应用专家论坛""中药材标准化基地考察及专家讲坛"等主题活动。南阳张仲景医药科技文化节是中医药产业发展成果的展示平台，也是中医药传统文化及其科技创新的推动弘扬的交流平台。

河南中医药大学仲景文化节是由河南中医药大学创办的，以突出其中原、中医、"仲景"办学特色的重要学术和文化活动，该活动以仲景艺术文化节和仲景学术文化节轮流为主题进行。

河南中医药大学仲景艺术文化节以"弘扬仲景文化，展示青春风采"为主题，结合高校中医药及相关专业大学生的专业学习和兴趣爱好，为学生们构建了一个学习交流仲景文化及展示自我、挑战自我的平台，得到了全校同学的广泛关注和积极参与，年均参与人数超过 30 000 人次。该艺术文化节主要包含各类仲景文体活动、艺术展演和中医药经典学术思想专家讲座等，如"感悟仲景·相约圣贤"朗读比赛、"习国学经典，传中华文化"中国传统文化挑战赛、"品读中医经典，共建健康中国"征文比赛、"仲景名师·名家面对面"讲座等活动。

河南中医药大学仲景学术文化节旨在宣传优良学术道德，浓厚仲景学术氛围，激发中医药师生的科研学术活力，促进仲景艺术和学术文化

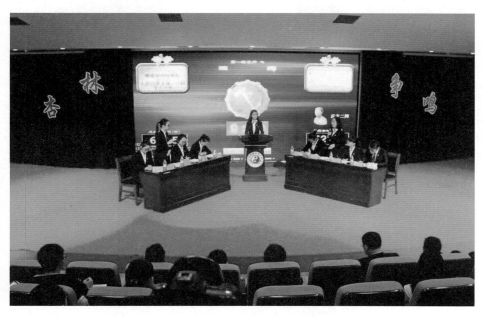

河南中医药大学第九届仲景文化节"杏林争鸣"辩论赛决赛
The final competition of the 9th Zhongjing Cultural Festival "Xinglin Controversy" Debate in Henan University of Chinese Medicine

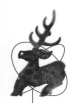

的传播和普及。该学术文化节主要包含"诵经典拜医圣""系列学术讲座""学术沙龙及国家基金申报和辅导""河南中医药大学科学技术协会会员代表大会""评选仲景学术思想传承与创新奖""仲景学术宣传及仲景文化宣讲""创新创业大赛"以及"仲景文化主题征文活动"等。

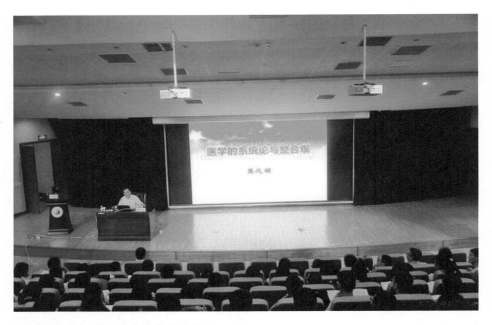

河南中医药大学仲景文化节学术讲座
Academic Lecture of Zhongjing Cultural Festival in Henan University of Chinese Medicine

Section Ⅴ   Zhongjing Culture Festival

Zhongjing Cultural Festival is an important way to "inherit Zhongjing's academic work and promote traditional Chinese medicine culture" in Henan and Nanyang. At present, the most famous cultural festival activities are

"Nanyang Zhang Zhongjing Medical Science and Technology Cultural Festival" and "Zhongjing Cultural Festival of Henan University of Chinese Medicine".

Nanyang Zhang Zhongjing Medical Science and Technology Cultural Festival, formerly known as Zhang Zhongjing Medical Culture Festival, started in 2002 and has been successfully held for 14 sessions by 2020. Nanyang Zhang Zhongjing Medical Science and Technology Cultural Festival is hosted by the Ministry of Science and Technology of the People's Republic of China, the State Administration of Traditional Chinese Medicine, and the People's Government of Henan Province. It aims to "inherit Zhongjing's academic work and carry forward the quintessence of traditional Chinese medicine". The themed activities mainly include "Traditional Chinese Medicine Science and Technology Innovation and Industrialization Development Strategy Forum", "Traditional Chinese Medicine Science and Technology Innovation and Industrialization Development Achievements Exhibition", "Traditional Chinese Medicine Culture Construction Seminar", "Zhang Zhongjing Classic Formula Application Expert Forum", "Investigation of the Standardization Base of Chinese Medicinal Materials and Expert Forum", and so on. This festival is an exchange platform to display the development achievements of traditional Chinese medicine industry, carry forward the excellent traditional culture of traditional Chinese medicine and promote its scientific and technological innovation.

Zhongjing Cultural Festival of Henan University of Chinese Medicine is an important academic and cultural activity founded by Henan University of Chinese Medicine to highlight its school-running characteristics of the Central Plains, traditional Chinese medicine, and "Zhongjing Academic". The event is themed around the "Zhongjing Art and Cultural Festival" and the "Zhongjing

195

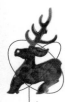

Academic and Cultural Festival".

The Zhongjing Art and Culture Festival of Henan University of Traditional Chinese Medicine creates a self-expression and self-challenge platform for students, as well as a platform for Zhongjing culture learning, This festival is under the theme of "promoting Zhongjing culture and showing youthful style", combining with the professional study and hobbies of college students majoring in traditional Chinese medicine and related majors. This event has received extensive attention and active participation of all students in the school, with an average annual number of participants exceeding 30,000. The festival mainly includes various kinds of cultural and sports activities, art exhibitions and academic lectures on traditional Chinese medicine classics, such as the reading competition of "Comprehend Zhongjing and Meet the Sages", the challenge competition of traditional Chinese culture of "Learn Classics and Spread Chinese Culture", the essay competition of "Read Chinese Medicine Classics and Build a Healthy China", "Famous Teachers and Masters Face to Face" lectures and other activities.

The Zhongjing Academic and Cultural festival of Henan University of Chinese Medicine aims to promote excellent academic ethics, enrich Zhongjing's academic atmosphere, stimulate the scientific research and academic vitality of teachers and students, and promote the dissemination and popularization of Zhongjing's art and academic culture. The academic and cultural festival mainly includes "Recite Classics and Worship Medical Saints", "Series of Academic Lectures", "Academic Salon and National Fund Declaration and Counseling", "Member Representative Meeting of Henan University of Traditional Chinese Medicine Science and Technology Association", "Selection of Zhongjing Academic Thought Inheritance and Innovation Award", "Zhongjing Academic Propaganda and Zhongjing Cultural

Propaganda", "Innovation and Entrepreneurship Competition" and "Theme Essay Activity on Zhongjing Culture".

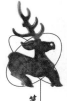

实践活动

1.参观河南中医药大学校史馆，体验"仲景文化节"相关艺术及学术活动。

2.观看体验南阳、河南中医药大学大学生仲景文化及艺术展演活动。

课后作业

1.对仲景文化的印象或看法，可以小组讨论。

2.完成一次仲景文化节相关活动的材料查询和收集。

Practical activities

1. Visit the College History Museum of Henan University of Chinese Medicine to experience the art and academic activities related to "Zhongjing Cultural Festival".

2. Watch and experience Zhongjing culture and art exhibition in Nanyang and Henan University of Chinese Medicine.

197

Homework

1. The impression or opinion of Zhongjing culture can be discussed in groups.

2. Complete the search and collection of materials related to one activity in Zhongjing Cultural Festival.